Women, Food,
and Diet in the Middle Ages

Women, Food, and Diet in the Middle Ages

Balancing the Humours

Theresa A. Vaughan

Routledge
Taylor & Francis Group
LONDON AND NEW YORK

First published in 2020 by Amsterdam University Press Ltd.

Published 2025 by Routledge
4 Park Square, Milton Park, Abingdon, Oxon OX14 4RN
605 Third Avenue, New York, NY 10158

Routledge is an imprint of the Taylor & Francis Group, an informa business

ISBN: 9789462989382 (hbk)
ISBN: 9781041190844 (pbk)
ISBN: 9781003709787 (ebk)
NUR 684

Cover illustration: "Giving Barley Soup to an Invalid", *Tacuinum Sanitatis*, SN2644, folio 44v; 1385-1390

Cover design: Coördesign, Leiden

DOI: 10.5117/9789462989382

For Product Safety Concerns and Information please contact our EU representative:
GPSR@taylorandfrancis.com
Taylor & Francis Verlag GmbH, Kaufingerstraße 24, 80331 München, Germany

For Kieran, my love

Table of Contents

List of Figures

Acknowledgments

There are a number of people who helped make this book possible. First, I would like to thank the University of Central Oklahoma for granting me sabbatical leave for the 2016-2017 school year. Having taken on a heavy service load for the previous twelve years, my sabbatical allowed me the chance to rebuild a research program and do some intensive research at the British Library and Bibliothèque nationale de France.

I would like to thank my dean, Catherine Webster, and department chairperson, Mark Silcox. Both of them not only helped me with logistics, but were both enthusiastic and encouraging about this project. Fellow faculty members in the Department of Humanities and Philosophy were also instrumental: Stephen C. Law, for so many things, not the least of which was encouraging me to do research in the medieval period in general and on foodways in particular; members of the departmental research and writing group, who generously read and commented upon a number of chapters – thank you Eva Dadlez, Mark Silcox, Joey Williams, Jerry Green, Reid Weber, Mary Brodnax, and Zach Norwood. Former dean Pam Washington was always buoyantly enthusiastic about my research projects, and numerous students stoically listened to me ramble on about medieval foodways – especially Beth Ussery, James Gregory, Mason Peck, Mason Werth, and Raven Wahkinney.

For whatever is good in this book, I owe a debt of gratitude to Henry Glassie, Dick Bauman, Gregory Schrempp, Beverly Stoeltje, Carol Greenhouse, Michael Herzfeld, and other graduate school professors who had probably given up on me writing my own book. I am also grateful for those who fought the battle of graduate school with me long ago, several of whom read the initial book proposal and offered helpful comments, especially John Laudun, Jason Baird Jackson, and Liz Locke.

Thanks to fellow members of the American Folklore Society Foodways Section, especially Diane Tye, Rachelle Saltzman, Mary Magoulick, Kristin McAndrews, LuAnne Roth, Lucy Long, Janet Gilmore, and Michael Owen Jones, who have known all along that foodways are a critical area of study. Inspirational members of the American Folklore Society Women's Section showed me very early in my career that women are a fascinating and worthwhile area of study – Jo Radner, Rosann Jordan, Kay Turner, and Amy Skillman all come to mind. And, of course, for Pauline Greenhill, the world's most productive folklorist, for graciously shepherding along past publications. I would also like to thank AUP editors Tyler Cloherty and

Shannon Cunningham for their support and encouragement, as well as careful reading and suggestions from reviewers who helped substantially improve this work. Mistakes and shortcomings are, it goes without saying, my own.

Finally, I could not have produced anything without the support of my family: Christopher Vaughan and Kathleen (O'Rourke) Vaughan, my parents, have always been enthusiastic cheerleaders for whatever I choose to do, not the least of which was this book. My children, Cian and Sam (Sarah) Mullen, put up with me being gone for extended periods during my sabbatical and then had to live with an often-distracted mother. Finally, Kieran Mullen, who has been my constant companion since 1988: husband, friend, confidante, proof-reader, fellow academic, and intellectual foil, he has always found a way to support my scholarly endeavours with energy and grace. It is to Kieran that I dedicate this book.

Introduction

Abstract
The introduction provides an overview of the research problems and how they will be approached, focusing particularly on how understanding women, food, medicine, and diet in the Middle Ages by using anthropological and folkloristic approaches can add to the understanding of these issues for non-elite populations. Research questions include: What do we know about women as food producers, feeders, and nurturers? What can be said about women as practitioners of folk or traditional medicine? How does this contrast with the written record of theoretical medicine? Finally, what were the cultural aspects surrounding women, food, and health, and how did it determine proper eating, fasting, and body shape?

Keywords: folk medicine, traditional medicine, medieval women, theoretical medicine

What can we know about women, food, and diet in the Middle Ages? Here, I cover a number of different interrelated topics having to do with medical dietary recommendations for women from the theoretical and practical medical traditions, the basis for those recommendations, and what we can learn about the folk traditions surrounding women, food and medicine. The book goes on to explore the themes of women and food more generally in the Middle Ages, with some parallels drawn with the Early Modern to contemporary issues involving diet, gendered roles in preparing and eating food, and medical views of women and food. Thus, this book is not exclusively about the medieval tradition of theoretical medicine and the role of food in medicine as it pertains to women. Instead, I seek to situate that tradition within the greater cultural context of women of all social classes, gendered expectations for women in gathering, preparing food, and feeding others, and the gaze on the female body and how it has been understood by the medical world as well as other quarters.

I write this book not as an historian, but rather as someone trained in both anthropology and folklore in the United States, with the particular

Vaughan, Theresa A., *Women, Food, and Diet in the Middle Ages: Balancing the Humours.* Taylor & Francis Group, 2020
DOI: 10.5117/9789462989382_INTRO

views of culture as a whole and folk culture that that education entails. Having spent most of my research career on gender and foodways, my turn to these subjects in the Middle Ages was as a result of establishing a teaching career in a field somewhat outside of my training: for the last twenty years I have taught in a department of Humanities and Philosophy, where I bring perspectives on both Western and non-Western cultures to students. Many of my departmental colleagues, from whom I have learned much over the years, are historians, art historians, archaeologists, classicists, philosophers, and those specializing in interdisciplinary humanities. My research career has been influenced by their focus on more conventional subjects in Western Civilization. I combine a curiosity for material and cultural artefacts with a focus on the subaltern – of those aspects of cultures and peoples that are part of the common person – of the folk, if you will.

In doing research on medieval foodways, I was struck by the fact that a number of the sources I read mentioned how little we know about women as cooks specifically, and how little we knew about women and food in general. The everyday lives of women who tended kitchen gardens, nursed children, and fed their families were not significant enough to have been recorded in any direct way. It is assumed, based upon the available evidence, that women's roles within the home as cooks and nurturers are fairly similar among the non-elite of many cultures. But what can we really know?

Food also formed the basis of the medieval healing system – of the humoral system as conceived by the Greeks – as a means to correct imbalance and maintain health. How did this pertain to women in particular? Could an understanding of women and food in the humoral system also tell us something about the nature of women and of their relationship to food? Interest in food, gender, and the humoral system led me to a better understanding of the expectations and restrictions placed on women's bodies in the Middle Ages. And, of course, none of this could be completely understood within its cultural context without some understanding of religion.

Essentially, what can we learn about women and food in the Middle Ages? That is my basic research question. I approach it through the lens of anthropology, but primarily through that of folklore studies. I rely on the work of historians, literary scholars, and archaeologists for source material and methods of approaching it. There are no new texts uncovered here; rather, I try to find a way of looking at existing information to see what we might be able to divine about women and foodways of all social strata.

To address the questions of women and food in the Middle Ages, this work explores a number of topics:

1 What do we know about women and food production?
2 What do we know about women as feeders and nurturers?
3 What do we know about women as practitioners of informal/traditional medicine?
4 How did theoretical medicine view the relationship between food and health, particularly as it pertained to women?
5 How did food appear in folk beliefs about women and health?
6 What were cultural expectations of women's bodies – both fed and abstinent?
7 How did cultural ideas about beauty and body size affect women's bodies?

Many of the medieval manuscripts on health have been identified, and a number have been studied in some depth. While I do not uncover any new texts nor suggest any heretofore undiscovered relationships between the various strands of medical learning, I hope this work adds to the academic conversation on medical texts by looking specifically at dietary recommendations for women's health, attempting to uncover both the humoral and cultural reasoning behind those recommendations. To accomplish this, I consider advice on diet and health from a number of sources. A brief look at contemporary cultural concerns about diet and health demonstrates that those same concerns, though framed differently, are present in medieval medicine. After all, we are all inheritors in one way or another of the Greek medical tradition, and Hippocrates' famous declaration, 'Let food be thy medicine, and medicine be thy food'.

However, looking at these texts still leaves us with many questions. Did medieval people follow this advice? Was it only intended for or followed by the aristocracy, who by the High Middle Ages could afford to hire academically trained doctors to prescribe diet and medicine for their health concerns? Did the advice for women in these guides become part of folk medicine, or the advice of traditional healers? Did folk medicine influence the written medical tradition?

Manuscripts here yield only limited evidence. The medieval manuscripts were written by the learned and literate. The writers themselves, depending upon the time period in question, came from the upper social strata – either trained in the ecclesiastical tradition, as clerics, or from the aristocracy and haute bourgeoisie. Literacy would, of course, eventually expand to other portions of the population, but the fact remains that we see folk culture and traditional learning mainly through the eyes of observers, rather than actors within that tradition.

The fields of folklore and anthropology have long grappled with understanding the traditions and practices of non-literate, non-hegemonic populations. While current trends in folklore and anthropology focus on the traditional cultures of living people, each field has a strong tradition of historical study as well, and of grappling with artefacts – be they material, verbal, or ritual – and expanding outward to understanding their place in a wider cultural field.

To offer a variety of approaches to this topic, I utilize a number of types of evidence and analyses. The goal here is to gather evidence from what we already know and look at it in a new light, to see what new things we can determine about the questions at hand. This is not to neglect the considerable work already done on the Middle Ages by historians, historical anthropologists, archaeologists, and literary scholars: this work would not be possible without all the groundwork achieved in these fields pertaining to food and health, as well as the experience of gender. Rather, this book builds on that earlier work.

In Chapter One, 'Women as Healers, Women as Food Producers', we look broadly at the role of women in many cultures as both the immediate providers of food, and of basic medical treatment for the family. In many cultures and time periods, women have been seen as the primary food providers and healers for the family, especially in non-aristocratic classes. Women's diets and food prepared by women carry unique symbolic meanings related to the role of women in society and in the family. An increasing array of literature on feminist approaches to foodways have helped to uncover women's work in the home and the symbolic and cultural load women carry in nurturing through food and healing. Some of that literature, I suggest, is particularly pertinent to the study of women's diet and health in the Middle Ages.

It can be difficult to truly view women's role as food providers and family healers in the medieval world. Long associated with domestic spaces in the Western world, women were less visible than men as public actors, and therefore their lives are less accessible to us. To complicate matters, most written records that come down to us from the medieval period were written almost exclusively by men. When focusing on medieval food and cuisine, we are faced with a relative abundance of written records, but again they are also primarily ecclesiastical and aristocratic. When literacy is confined to those two groups, it is logical that most written accounts will be from and about those groups. If we want to look closely at women and food in the Middle Ages – women as cooks, managers of the domestic space, food vendors, and as consumers, we are hindered by the availability of material as well. There is an abundance of evidence for food production and consumption among the aristocracy, but if we wish to look at women as cooks, we are thwarted even within the aristocratic class, as the grand kitchens of the aristocracy were run and staffed almost exclusively by men. Ecclesiastical writing, aside from records of purchase and consumption by convents and monasteries, view food through the lens of Christian teachings on abstinence and avoidance of gluttony, also associating food with sexuality. Such writing is nearly always prescriptive rather than descriptive.

So, what can we learn about women and food in the Middle Ages, especially beyond the convent or the manor house? Positive examples can be found in, for example, conduct literature; negative examples appear in genres such as the fabliau. This chapter addresses some of the literature on women as consumers and producers of food, with implications for understanding the cultural significance of diet and women's health in the Middle Ages.

In Chapter Two, 'Medieval Theories of Nutrition and Health', the two threads of Greek medicine are examined for their insights into how the body uses food and gender differences in the way food was processed, with emphasis on the Hippocratic tradition as seen in Galen. An understanding of humoral theory, on which much medieval medicine was based, is necessary to follow the arguments of later medical writers about how food influences health, and what food is recommended both for the maintenance of good health and the treatment of disease. Humoral theory also explains how diet is often related to disease, and how dietary remedies can help cure various medical conditions. This chapter also covers some of the trends and modifications to humoral theory made during the medieval period.

While humoral theory is often complex, this brief overview necessitates some simplification. An emphasis on the differences in dietary needs by age, gender, and state of health is explored to better understand why certain dietary recommendations were made specifically for women's health. While most medieval medical authors had access to the same texts or copies of texts, those texts may have been fragmentary, corrupted, or incomplete. Changes in medical theory, particularly beginning with the establishment of medical schools in the 1100s, are also apparent in medical texts. The arrival of systemized and translated Arabic texts, themselves drawn largely from the medicine of ancient Greece, also changed the medical landscape. However, most of the work addressed in this book is ultimately traced back to the original Greek ideas of diet and health.

In Chapter Three, 'The Special Problem of Nutrition and Women's Health', we move beyond general humoral theory to those texts which spend at least some time talking about health concerns specific to women. Medieval literature on women's medicine is relatively scarce; how then do we understand recommendations and practices specific to women? The *Trotula* was a foundational text, cited for several hundred years. Women's health was mentioned occasionally in other medical texts: I emphasize Hildegard of Bingen as a female author working within both the theological and medical traditions. These texts are examined within the context of humoral theory. While both the *Trotula* and the works of Hildegard are addressed in much greater detail in Chapter Five, they're included here as part of a textual tradition on women's health.

A survey of medical texts, and those on natural philosophy focusing on reproduction and female anatomy, helps to understand how the female body was viewed from several different vantage points – humoral theory certainly, but also anatomy and, surprisingly for contemporary readers, theology. What was it about the nature of the female being that made it prone to certain illnesses? Here, again, we see Greek ideas wend their way through the medieval tradition – sometimes strikingly misogynous in tone. Humoral theory was sometimes used to justify anti-feminist medical viewpoints. Female bodies were weaker than male bodies; more delicate and prone to certain illnesses. Pregnancy, a condition unique to women, was viewed as a natural state, but one in which the body should be treated as if it were ill. Often, dietary recommendations for the ill or recuperated are reflected in those recommendations for pregnant women.

Chapter Four, 'Theoretical Medicine vs. Practical Medicine', investigates the problems of separating medicine as written and presumably practiced by academically trained physicians from more common remedies used by local healers, midwives, and wise women. A distinction must be made between the theoretical medicine of academically trained doctors and the practical medicine of midwives and traditional healers, perhaps better classified as 'folk medicine' or 'traditional medicine'. Historians have studied the changing role and status of traditionally trained midwives. In the later Middle Ages, midwives were partially displaced by academically trained doctors for both the aristocracy and the bourgeoise. While the extent to which midwives were supplanted by male doctors may have been overstated, the rise of medical schools and of academically trained physicians did cause change in the medical landscape.

The practical medicine of midwives and traditional healers is, of course, more difficult to document as it was not primarily a written tradition. Some traces of it may exist in the *Trotula*. Some may be found in other kinds of records, folktales, legal proceedings, trials for heresy, herbals and other illuminated manuscripts, and in fragmentary ways in a number of sources. We know quite a bit about folk medicine in a number of contemporary cultures – how much of what we know may be applicable to the fragmentary evidence from the Middle Ages?

Chapter Five, 'The *Trotula* and the Works of Hildegard of Bingen', offers a more thorough examination of the most common medieval text about women's gynaecological and reproductive health, in part with the aim of trying to understand how these works might be related to folk medicine. The *Trotula*, traditionally attributed to a female author, is examined as an historical document and a possible record of both theoretical and practical medicine in twelfth century Salerno. The *Trotula* itself, really three different texts that explore aspects of women's health, cosmetics, and beauty, is in reality only partially written by a woman or her students. However, its importance as an authoritative text attributed to a woman cannot be overemphasized. The portion that may have been written by Trota or her students is, in fact, more practical and less theoretical than the other two parts. Can this offer us some insight into folk medicine, at least in Salerno and surrounding regions?

Within the *Trotula*, dietary recommendations offer us a look into the role diet was thought to play in women's health. Some of its recommendations are analysed within the framework of humoral theory. Is it possible to determine which dietary recommendations were theoretically determined by humoral theory, and which may have come from folk medicine? To what extent did humoral theory reach the understanding of diet among the common people? It is impossible to know the answers to these questions with certainty, but literature on folk medicine and traditional healing may help to sort out some of the text, and provide suggestions for areas of further inquiry.

We also take a look at an author whose recommendations existed outside of mainstream theoretical medicine. In contrast to the *Trotula*, Hildegard of Bingen's texts addressed medicine and natural philosophy through a highly idiosyncratic theoretical framework. The two relevant books, among the many written by Hildegard (or at least attributed to her), are entitled *Physica* and what has come to be called *Causae et Curae*.

Hildegard's works are not exclusively focused on women's health and reproduction, but they do address these topics within a theological framework that treats understanding the body as a microcosm of God's creation. Here, they are examined for instructions on women's health, and particularly for dietary recommendations specific to women and reproductive health. How much of Hildegard's recommendations reflect her knowledge of folk medicine and traditional healing, and how much are they simply reflective of her own brand of theology? Do they offer a window into the larger culture of diet and health in Germany of the 1100s, or are they simply cut from the cloth of Hildegard's imagination? There is no doubt that Hildegard's mind was sharp and expansive, as she wrote on so many subjects, but she was also a person of a specific time and culture. It is conceivable that traditional medicine is found in her recommendations.

In Chapter Six, 'The Legacy of the *Trotula*', we look more closely at the *Trotula*'s influence on later texts, and textual traditions that existed apart from the *Trotula* and its legacy. An examination of other texts that address diet and health, particularly women's health, reveals how interpretation of the *Trotula* evolved over time, as understanding of diet and health evolved. By the fifteenth century, ideas springing from humoral theory were still present, but as more people became literate, general guides for understanding of animals, plants, and spices and their properties became popular among the aristocracy and haute bourgeoisie.

Of key interest are the various versions of the *Regimen sanatitis* produced in the fourteenth and fifteenth centuries. While not specifically focused on women's health, they did feature diet, health, and to some extent, cooking. Platina's *On Right Pleasure and Good Health* is another example of an author building upon both medical theory (as it came to be understood by learned lay people) and *Regimina sanitatis* and their careful descriptions of all things edible to recommend what he considered to be the best medical practices. These texts are examined for dietary recommendations most pertinent to women and women's concerns. Finally, late texts addressing women's health, such as Michele Savonarola's *Regimine pregnantium*, and pseudo-medical texts, such as *De secretis mulierum,* analyze diet and women's health recommendations through the misogynistic lens of men whose view of women was particularly problematic.

In Chapter Seven, 'Women's Diets and Standards of Beauty', we look at not just the recommendations for good health and the amelioration of gynaecological heath issues, but also how dietary recommendations for women were connected to standards of beauty. What role did diet play in expectations for women's beauty and attractiveness? How did the expectations for the appearance of a women's body relate to her weight? Were obesity's effects on beauty as well as health similar to current standards? Evidence suggests that until the later Middle Ages, obesity was not necessarily viewed as an aesthetic problem, but was viewed morally as indicative of a lack of self-control and indulgence in the sin of gluttony. By the Early Modern period, it was also of great concern as an impediment to fertility. How does this manifest (or does it manifest) in the medical texts, both for women's health in particular and general recommendations on diet? In this case, works on the anthropology of the body suggest that what women eat and how they look are deeply embedded social constructs revealing cultural attitudes towards gender difference, women's roles, and worth.

Chapter Eight, 'Religious Conflict and Religious Accommodation', addresses the role played by Church teachings against gluttony and on the inherently sinful nature of women in dietary recommendations for health. The Church had much to say about the virtues of fasting and meat avoidance in the spiritual health of both men and women. The conflict between recommendations for bodily health and spiritual health is examined, highlighting the sometimes-uneasy compromise between medical and ecclesiastical dietary recommendations, particularly for women.

The works of Hildegard are especially important in observing one synthesis between the two points of view. In addition, texts such as *De secretis mulierum* by Pseudo-Albertus Magnus, first introduced in Chapter Six and steeped in the anti-feminist tradition, are instructive in showing the extent to which Church attitudes could be at odds with the more neutral stance of medical texts. As we have seen, anti-feminist traditions in the area of women's health and physiology go all the way back to ancient Greece, but the concept of sin fed directly into such phenomena as holy anorexia, self-denial, and endurance of illness as a form of self-mortification.

The final chapter, Chapter Nine, is entitled 'Evolving Advice for Women's Health Through Diet'. It provides a summary overview of how dietary advice for women changed from Galen through the Early Modern period, and anticipates some of the changes taking place in dietary recommendations during the Renaissance and beyond. While this is a long arc of history, certain trends can be traced. The literature from folklore and anthropology will also prove useful here. How do cultural attitudes towards diet change?

A summary of the main arguments and findings of the previous chapters places humoral theory and its dietary implications within the context of other global dietary theories and practices. What can other cultures in other contexts tell us about informal learning of foodways, changes in traditional medicine, modified roles for women, and popular religion as it relates to food culture?

Ultimately, examining the interrelationship between medicine, health, nurturing, sexuality, and women's bodies may lead to new ways of looking at or understanding women's lives and bodies in the Middle Ages. Looking at both the culture of the elite and the non-elite may also inspire new attempts to understand the traditional, informal culture of diet and medicine alluded to by some medical and non-medical texts.

Cultural attitudes toward health and illness, toward food and cuisine, toward women and female bodies always inform and underlie texts that purport to be scientific and medical. Each text is written within a nested series of cultural assumptions, some clearly evident, others less so. People who were not part of the literate tradition had as distinct and coherent a culture as did those of the literate classes; attitudes toward women and health are also present there, even if we can understand them only imperfectly.

1 Women as Healers, Women as Food Producers

Abstract
Women have served as providers of food and basic medical care for their families both in the European Middle Ages and worldwide, especially for the majority of people who do not have the means to hire either a physician or servants. These roles have significant symbolic meanings within cultures. Uncovering the reality of women in domestic spaces in the Middle Ages has its challenges, especially for the lower classes, for reliable information is scarce. The everyday lives of women were not typically thought important enough to document. A look at a variety of textual and non-textual evidence through the lens of the disciplines of folklore and anthropology can help suggest interpretations which fill in some of the gaps in our knowledge.

Keywords: foodways, anthropology of food, medieval women, domestic spaces

The preparation of food is an intimate act, as is feeding others. Women are the first food providers we know. The act of feeding from the breast was and is normal, and provides an infant with its first sustenance. To medieval people, breastfeeding would have been a common, everyday sight. It was also lauded in images of the lactating Virgin – *Maria lactans* – Mary feeding the infant Jesus. From then on women, as far as we can tell, were the primary food providers in the families of common people. It is not until we reach the level of the aristocracy, or in later medieval times, the haute bourgeoise, that we begin to see cooking become the province of professional male cooks. The majority of people were fed by a wife, mother, or other women if the food they ate was prepared in the home. In some places, such as England, women also provided the drink (Vaughan 2011). Food was and is one area in which women had power within the family. Sometimes that power was

Vaughan, Theresa A., *Women, Food, and Diet in the Middle Ages: Balancing the Humours.* Taylor & Francis Group, 2020
DOI: 10.5117/9789462989382_CH01

seized and acted upon in a refusal to eat – such was the case with 'holy anorexia' – most clearly explained by Carol Walker Bynum (1987). Women eating are sometimes shown in artwork, occasionally reported in tales, but more frequently framed in terms of gluttony: women and men eating too much. The Church steadily preached against gluttony, morality plays and didactic writing warned of its danger (Knight 1983; Vigarello 2010). Fabliaux, bawdy French stories of the 1200s, often used women and eating to allude to sexuality (Gordon 2007). The Church, in fact, thought overeating was a 'gateway sin' leading to other occasions of sin, such as fornication. Women who were associated with food and drink in public places, such as taverns, were also often linked with unbridled sexuality. Women fed, but they also ate.

An abundance of literature in multiple disciplines points out the importance of women as food producers; some address the idea of women as healers, and some cover the intersection of both. This first chapter offers an overview of women as healers and food producers, concentrating on women in the folk or common culture. Are there approaches and theoretical stances drawn from contemporary anthropological and folkloristic approaches which could enhance our understanding of medieval women, diet, and health? First, a brief overview of the fields of folklore and anthropology and their potential contributions to understanding these aspects of medieval foodways and healing as they pertain to women.

Folklore, a form of academic study more historically focused than the related field of anthropology, places artefacts themselves at the centre of study. That artefact may be a belief, tale, material object, custom, or any one of a number of manifestations of informal, traditional culture. Investigating that object, the folklorist details its features and characteristics, then expands outward to include everything it is possible to know about its context, performance, and intended audience. Theoretical approaches that reach beyond the descriptive can enhance understanding of that artefact and its culture of origin – functional, structural, Marxist, post-modern, diachronic and synchronic, phenomenological, semiotic, and other theoretical orientations have all been used. Historically, however, folklore began as the impulse to collect songs, stories, and beliefs of the European peasantry as early as the late eighteenth century.

John Lindow has recently argued that, in fact, the study of medieval texts and the study of folklore grew out of the same impulse, and had the same origins. While textual study of manuscripts has gone in various directions since the 1800s, the folkloristic approach brings to bear ideas of performativity, flexibility and process of traditions, and an understanding of the fluid relationship between oral and literate forms (Lindow 2018). Folklore was born out of Romantic Nationalism, as was the case in continental Europe or Ireland, or out of social evolutionary theories that made folklore out to be the relic of a barbarian past still present in the lower classes, as in England.

Folkloristic approaches to foodways, whether historical or contemporary, have tended to focus on food and identity – sometimes personal identity, but more often the ways in which group identity is negotiated and reified through the making and sharing of food. In addition, there has been research on food and gender – both as a site of transmission of the informal culture held among women, and as a point of resistance to restrictive gender roles and negotiation of family identity and expectations. Foodways also intersect with what folklorists would call folk belief, as well as folk medicine. Women, who often hold the role of family healer and first line treatment of illness, have long passed on knowledge of basic herblore and traditional remedies. They are also the providers of food within the family.

Both food preparation and home medical treatment are wrapped up in the ideas of care, particularly the sometimes-invisible work that women undertake within the family. For contemporary cultures, folklorists and anthropologists have undertaken in fieldwork to better understand women as food providers and healers. Interviews with women became more frequent, as both fields realized the ubiquitous focus on strictly male aspects of culture in place until the 1970s. Anthropological approaches, which can take many forms, have drawn upon nutritional evidence, development, political implications, centring the idea of agency, symbolic analysis, and other approaches (Mintz and Du Bois 2002; Klein and Watson 2016). Identity is one among them. Folkloristic approaches have tended to place identity, agency, and the actual material culture at their centre.

According to Lucy Long, a folklorist who has spent much of her career writing and thinking about foodways,

> [Ethnographic tradition in folklore] insists on understanding meanings as personally as well as socially constructed and on interpreting these meanings as the result of individual choices elected from a range of cultural options. This approach to meaning acknowledges that the political – issues of power, hierarchy, and status – shapes the options available to individuals and the choices that they make. Folklorists have historically tended to focus on the connectedness created by traditions and community, whether those communities are the geographically and culturally bounded ones of the stereotypical or the looser, more fluid ones of postmodern society (2009, 6).

Long also argues that, while the field of folklore has been accused of being overly romantic in its views, its central focus on the creative products of human culture (such as food) give a nexus from which to examine interlocking threads of expression – a food product is tied to multiple genres and meanings. This approach was taken by some of the first in the field of folklore; for example, in 1972 Don Yoder described foodways, which he termed 'Folk Cookery', as the centre of multiple strands of aesthetics and genre, in a plea to bring it under the umbrella of what was then termed 'folklife'. This was part of a larger movement to study folklife – the practices of a group – rather than to simply concentrate on oral genres (Long 2015).

Some examples of ways in which folklorists (as well as others) use foodways as a nexus of multivalent meaning are: intergenerational contact, questions of gender and identity, the relationship to legends or beliefs about the dish or the component foodstuffs, culturally-bound knowledge about how to treat or process the food for best effect, any medicinal uses for that food, ideas of what food promotes health, rituals which should be undertaken before or while making the food, gender rules about who can or should prepare the food, taboos about who or how one can have contact with food, and a myriad of other elements (Jones 2007). Most of this can be uncovered and deciphered through the use of fieldwork on contemporary communities, but also by examining historical documents such as cookbooks, personal recipe collections, photos, and resources such as the food collections from the WPA Archives. But this is all a question of methodology, rather than theory. Diane Tye (2010) uses the written record, her mother's collection of recipes, as a focal point for tracing her mother's life history, and examining her own relationship to that history. Janet Theophano, another folklorist, looks more broadly at cookbooks for what they can tell us about women's lives (2002). Theoretical approaches to folklore study have tended to come to the field through anthropology and literary studies.

Anthropological approaches

Anthropology began its life as a part of the colonial endeavour. Anthropologists sought to understand what it deemed 'primitive' peoples, primarily encountered in areas occupied by colonial powers, as this is where Euro-American students of culture had the most contact. Eventually the field developed the method of 'participant observation', a method of studying people by living among them, learning their language (ideally), and experiencing their customs first-hand. While participant observation has been the gold standard in the field for quite some time, synchronic analysis has made room for diachronic analysis as well. One critique of anthropology is that it has treated peoples it has studied as having no history, of existing in an ever-present and unchanging now. Anthropology as a field has responded to that critique by becoming more attentive to history. American anthropology of the 1980s took a more visible historic turn, exhibited in such classic works as Eric Wolf's *Europe and the People Without History* (1982), and *Sweetness and Power* by Sidney Mintz (1985). A different approach arose in France, developing out of the *Annales* School. This school of history was one of the first to employ methodologies that examined daily life, economics, and culture. Food became an element of the study of history in the interwar years as France and then other European schools of historical study began to shift focus to societal influences on history. The *Annales* school was, for example, the first historical school to seriously look at food history. Some current descendants of this school acknowledge the specifically anthropological approach to history now called "historical anthropology". The Annales school focused on history's *longue durée* – or the long view, of the history of common people and their culture – which changed more slowly than the story of military history, of the lives of royalty, and other areas of more interest to traditional historical discourse.

From French historical anthropology we get historical methodology applied to understanding common people. Authors such as Leroy La Durie, Jacques Le Goff, Phillip Ariès, and later Jean-Louis Flandrin, Jean-Claude Schmidtt, and historians outside of France, most notably Massimo Montanari, were concerned specifically with the Middle Ages (Watts 2012). Each has brought to bear some of the intellectual traditions of anthropology with the methodology of history to better understand medieval people and their lives. Sometimes, a written record exists which records the worldview of an individual, such as in the book *The Cheese and the Worms* by Carlo Ginzburg (1992 [1980]). Sometimes it is an assembly of information from many sources which gives some idea of how the common people, the silent people of history, lived their lives. What were the rhythms of the year? What was daily life like? How can we tell? Sometimes written records are available, but must be interpreted within the framework of the culture.

So, what does an anthropological approach add to the study of history? First, as mentioned above, an inclination towards understanding the lives of common people. There have, of course, been plenty of historians who have sought to understand aspects of this, and more frequently in the later twentieth century than in the early part of the century. But anthropologists want to understand not just events, records, and other documentable things, they want to understand the culture of the people. Culture itself is challenging to define well. As Alfred Kroeber, key American anthropologist of the twentieth century wrote, 'What culture is can be better understood from knowledge of what forms it takes and how it works than by definition' (1987 [1952], p. 80). Culture includes speech, knowledge, belief, art, morality, customs, worldview, technologies, and other aspects of social life that are informally learned and implicit in social interactions. Understanding culture provides us with a way of making sense of social life and the ability to construct identity. It is the background against which all action takes place.

This focus on the cultural can enrich historical understanding by making plain unspoken assumptions which lie behind the actions deemed sufficiently important to have been recorded. Anthropologists who have taken to understanding food systems, for example, are often focused not just on what people eat, but how it is acquired or grown, how much people need to eat to maintain minimum caloric requirements, how crops are domesticated and the technology of cultivation, and what systems of trade operate so that groups have access to food not grown or processed in the area. Anthropologists studying food systems also look at who prepares food, and the symbolic meaning of the preparation, serving, and eating of food for members of a culture. In the case of this study, historical anthropology helps us to understand what food was required to maintain health, how it was processed, and what the food may mean symbolically.

While anthropological and folkloristic perspectives are related in many ways, there are also differences in the way they approach the interpretation of food preparation and consumption. The folklorist, as shown above, is more likely to take cooking as part of a cultural or ethnic tradition, and focus on the act of preparation and eating as enactments of identity. Anthropologists, while not necessarily discounting those approaches, tend to look at cooking and eating in terms of larger cultural patterns and food systems, at least in more recent work. Anthropologists have approached food taboos, for example, in terms of cultural materialism (Harris 1998 [1985]), symbolic analysis (Douglas 1975), structuralism (Lévi-Strauss 1966), Marxism (Mintz 1985), and ritual analysis (Fox 2014). Likewise, medical anthropology intersects with the anthropology of food and eating where food is viewed as curative or edible plants are used to make medicines.

Work on medieval foodways done by archaeologists has been able to provide us with specifics as to what was consumed, how much, how it changed over time, how it was stored and prepared, and how actual preparation and consumption may have differed from the appearance of food preparation and consumption in other sources, whether in literature, stories, cookbooks, illustrations, proverbs, or other means (Gazin-Schwartz and Holtorf 1999). For example, written and visual sources can tell us what was valued and what food was higher in status. Early recipe collections can tell us how this ideal food would have been prepared. Epics that include feasting convey the importance of abundance and the status of individual foods (Poor and Schulman 2007). Archaeology can provide information about what food was actually consumed – through the analysis of physical remains of bones, ethnobotany, physical layouts of kitchens, and so forth. Sometimes archaeological results contradict the idealized form of cooking and eating conveyed in other sources, and that knowledge is important (Woolgar, Serjeantson, and Waldron 2009).

Archaeology has also been used to try to determine what spaces in the medieval household served as gendered spaces, or whether in fact there were gendered spaces (Gilchrist 1999). Are our ideas about women as cooks (at least in non-aristocratic or non-wealthy families) accurate? How can we tell? Is there a way to tell the difference between what women and men ate, in terms of archaeological evidence? Not all of these questions have been answered, but the work of archaeologists holds promise for advancing our understanding of gender and material culture in the Middle Ages[1].

The sometimes questionable agenda of both anthropology and folklore studies, whether the colonial enterprise or the romanticization of the rural peasant, has clouded the conclusions of scholars. However, both fields as they exist in the United States have largely moved beyond their often-problematic origins, with anthropologists now studying both Western and non-Western cultures, and folklorists moving beyond the culture of Europe into a more global perspective. The two fields often share similar theoretical orientations.

However, each field does retain its own distinct identity. Anthropology is clearly a social science, with all that implies. In the United States, four subfields are contained under one discipline: cultural anthropology, linguistic anthropology, archaeology, and biological anthropology. In Europe, the subfields operate much more independently. Historical archaeology is another field that often operates independently. Folklore, however, while

1 Please note, I am including a discussion of the contributions of archaeology under the heading of anthropology. In the United States, anthropology is a four-field discipline, including cultural anthropology – my home discipline – linguistic anthropology, biological anthropology, and archeology. In Europe, these fields tend to be separate. There is also a difference between historical archaeology – taught by history departments – and those doing prehistorical anthropology – usually trained as anthropologists. The two fields are, of course, related, and anthropological archeology can examine historical topics.

present both in Europe and in the United States, still retains elements of Romantic Nationalism in Europe. It has played a more minor role in American folklore study due to the lack of a long-standing peasantry and no need to recover a lost identity, but rather to forge a new one. The field of folklore also exists as a discipline which straddles two large types of inquiry: social science, and humanities. Folklore reaches out to both anthropology and literary studies equally, and its history is interwoven with each.

Both fields can help us understand what is happening on the ground, among common people. Investigations into food culture are common to both fields. Together, they address not only what was eaten and how it was prepared, but also its symbolic meanings, role in social relationships, changes that reflect shifting cultural elements, gender divisions, social customs, religious significance, and role in identity. In addition, each field also has a history of inquiry into traditional healing and traditional remedies, as well as all the cultural elements surrounding them. Each approach will help to better understand food and health in the Middle Ages, not only from the point of view of literate and professional writers of medical texts, but also of the common people.

Other ways of knowing are also important. Food Studies, by its very nature, is interdisciplinary. It is often paired with the fields of nutrition, medicine, economics, archaeology, history, anthropology, feminist studies, and folklore, among others. 'Common among these works is the notion that studying the most banal of human activities can yield crucial information and insights about both daily life and world view, from what is in the pot to the significance of the fire that heats it' (Avakian and Haber 2005, 2).

We cannot seriously consider foodways without understanding the crucial role that women have played in the provisioning and cooking of food for the vast majority of people. Often absent in the medieval literature, overshadowed by the aristocratic cooking traditions of their male cooks and authors, a feminist perspective is another way to understand what is often hidden behind the literate and aristocratic evidence.

Work by medievalists

There has been quite a lot of work done by medievalists on medicine (primarily through medical texts), food (from a variety of viewpoints), and gender (also from a variety of viewpoints). While there is not an overabundance of information on the intersection of these three topics (with the possible exception of medicine and gender), there is work that can be utilized or combined. Medieval Studies is an interdisciplinary field itself, with a variety of approaches used in understanding the materials available to us, whether they be texts, art, or material evidence. Historians, linguists, literary scholars, theologians, and those in religious studies, have all tended to focus primarily on the textual tradition. More than two hundred years of careful work has been done in manuscript studies, examination of court and manorial records, and a variety of other texts existing from this time period. Texts of various kinds, of course, provide a deep well of information from which to draw. Much of the work done on the Western Middle Ages has been done using textual information. In the area of women and health, for example, the careful textual study of Monica Green (c.f. [2002 and 2008]) is instrumental in tracing the influence of the *Trotula*, the position of women in the medical field, and other areas pertinent to this study. Other scholars have done significant work on women and medicine into the early modern period: King 2007, Evans 2014, Toulalan 2017, and Cabré 2000. Others have looked closely at food and cuisine: c.f. Henisch 1990 [1976] , Jacquart 2006, Laurioux 2002, Montanari 2012, Nicoud 2006, and Scully 1995.

The work of those who have closely read texts and helped uncover the textual tradition are, of course, invaluable in this study. While I make use of the historical work, my interpretation is necessarily that of a folklorist with a background in anthropology.

How can we approach medieval sources?

Looking at women in the kitchen through the lens of power versus subjugation, medievalists do not agree on how to interpret the somewhat circumscribed role of women. To a large extent, the lives of aristocratic women were more strictly regulated than those of non-aristocratic women, although these women certainly enjoyed access to greater wealth and in some notable instances, power (Pernoud 1998). Some earlier work by medievalists on women tended to focus on their victimization in a highly hierarchical, patriarchal, and Church-controlled society. Later work has focused more on the agency of medieval women, and their ability to work to their own advantage within the strictures of social norms. Some have suggested that women's influence within the domestic sphere was empowering:

> Returning to the question of the household, it can be suggested that women had greater competency within the house and its material culture than men and therefore may have experienced a sense of greater power

> and the possibility of agency in the sense of 'power-to' rather than 'power-over' other members of the household (Smith 2007a, 313).

Others argue that women might have had limited power in the kitchen because the cooks of great households were all men, and that the early modern period brought a change which allowed women access to both literate culture in the writing of cookbooks, and in changing social roles, bringing women more influence in the realm of cuisine (van Winter 2007).

The question of diet and women's health in the Middle Ages certainly relies upon textual evidence – as any historian would agree – but also on other kinds of evidence. Archaeological explorations of medieval diet (for example [Woolgar, Serjeantson, and Waldron 2009]) gives us some idea of the material culture involved in the preparation of food, as well as definitive evidence for what type of food was consumed. When looking strictly at material culture, archaeology tells us much about the kinds of cooking utensils commonly used, where the fire was placed, and what methods of cooking were employed by medieval people. Medieval illustrations help confirm or add information to the archaeological findings. Coroner's rolls tell us about the dangers of household tasks for women and children, including cooking (Hanawalt 1986). Legal records demonstrate that women were interested in retaining power over their property, ran small food-oriented businesses, and likewise were apt to use the legal system to their own benefit, or could be fined for not following local food regulations. Medieval medicine reveals how the medical experts adapted Greek, Arab, and Jewish learning to prescribe how women, especially aristocratic women, should eat (Caballero-Navas 2008). We know from ecclesiastical writings that gluttony was condemned and that women were associated with sexuality: sexuality was associated with gluttony (Vigarello 2010). A study of hagiography tells us that some women rejected food (and denied sexuality) as a means to spiritual and social power (Espi-Forcen 2012). Didactic treatises from the later medieval period offer instructions for how and what to cook, and reveal the role of women in the managing of the kitchen (Greco and Rose 2009). Various kinds of folklore reveal expectations of women in the realm of food, cautions against straying from gender norms, and the inversion of gender norms that medieval people seem to have found amusing (Crocker 2006). Many sources tell us about class differences in both eating and cooking, and, unfortunately, tell us much more about the aristocratic class than the peasant. Taken together, this diverse work can create some understanding of women and food in the Middle Ages.

Women as healers

Although relatively rare, especially among professional physicians, it certainly was not impossible for women to be recognized as healers, even in the written tradition (a topic examined in detail in later chapters). And, of course, healing went far beyond the work of university-trained physicians. How do we define healing? Is it the administration of herbs or other substances serving as medicine? Is it the knowledge of surgery or the setting of bones? Is it knowing the right prayers and charms to heal? Does it lie in prescribing the proper diet to ameliorate a condition? Is it knowing how to help a labouring woman deliver a baby? Is healing dedicated nursing care, or attending to the needs of one who is ill? Of course, it can be all of these things. The point, of course, is that one does not need to have received a university education to serve as a healer.

Informal medical knowledge was, and still is, passed along traditionally – from learning to care for the sick by watching a family member attend to another's comfort during illness, to knowing basic herblore and preparation of beneficial substances from those herbs. Traditional learning can teach the basics of recognizing disease to knowing how a person should be fed during illness. Even today, we all learn some of the basics of care and treatment from family members, from the way a parent cleans and dresses a wound, to a mother's hands telling her when a child has a fever. Folk medicine – the traditional medicine of the people – is a realm of informal knowledge in which we all participate to varying degrees (Brady 2001). In the Middle Ages, this would certainly have been true. Oral transmission, after all, is one of the hallmarks of folk medicine, and would have been the only form of learning available to the majority of people, who were illiterate. As we come to the close of the Middle Ages, more books of health become available to a lay audience (such as the various *Regimina sanitatis*), but for most people, oral transmission and observation were the primary teachers.

About four hundred different plant species were known in Western Europe. There were, of course, apothecaries and doctors versed in herblore, but so were wise women and traditional female healers. While some of the knowledge of the uses of these herbs and simples was retained in leech books or other medical resources listing medical treatments by disease, there were also herbals, such as Galen's Herbal (Everett 2014) or the Carrera Herbal (Kyle 2017), which listed herbs in order, noting their uses. The difference was in the arrangement of the information (Stannard 2013). While few women would have had access to these texts, or would have known how to read them in the first place, much of medical lore was passed down orally. That lore might include some herbal remedies, as well as knowledge of certain foods and their treatment in ailments. 'Some plants, for example, were valued as primary foodstuffs – wheat and barley, naturally, but also cabbage and radish plus a number of fruits and nuts, for example, apples and quinces, hazel nuts and chestnuts' (Stannard 2013, 48). While the nutritional value of each foodstuff might have been known through some dissemination of humoral theory or simply recommendations from authoritative sources, the use of these items as traditional medicines was also known. Sometimes herbs themselves were used primarily for flavour, but at least twenty-five common medieval herbs continued to be used in traditional medicine long after the Middle Ages (Stannard 2013). Outside of the realm of apothecaries and physicians, a knowledge of some herbs and basic traditional remedies would have been common among most women versed in the folk tradition.

Women today are still considered the primary loci of informal comfort and healing within families (Cabré 2008). Commercials aimed at 'Doctor Mom' play on the idea that women's roles as nurturers include providing basic medical care and comfort to their families. Perhaps this derives from the amount of time she shares with her family, being the primary person to stay up with a sick child or care for aging parents, or is a cultural outgrowth of the time spent raising infants and small children. That doesn't preclude men from taking on this role, of course, but our cultural expectation is that women are more likely to serve as the family healer.

Was the situation the same in the Middle Ages? It is known that monasteries for both men and women contained infirmaries, with at least one monk or nun assuming the role of caregiver. Hildegard of Bingen, discussed in Chapter Five, may have been one such woman. The aristocrat was able to consult more formally trained healers, either formal physicians, apothecaries, or surgeons. These would more likely have been male, although there is some indication that women in labour were still attended by other women, if depictions and descriptions are accurate (Bavaye-Kouidrat 2016). For the peasant woman or village dweller, an apothecary or barber-surgeon could be consulted if the family had the means, but it was more likely that women served as the primary caregivers and healers. Certainly, during childbirth, it was women who attended the birth, perhaps with the aid of a locally recognized midwife or wise woman, someone with the training of experience, or perhaps apprenticeship to another midwife. Although this would change to some extent during the Early Modern period, women were still the most commonly found in the birthing chamber.

It was also likely that women provided comfort and nursing care to family members, or perhaps neighbours or extended family who needed attending during illness (Cabré 2008). Some written works, such as the *Distaff Gospels* (Garay and Jeay 2006), a humorous text in the anti-feminist tradition intended for an aristocratic audience, inadvertently demonstrate that women would have been versed in oral lore pertaining to healing. Whether or not remedies were effective by modern standards is immaterial, as they helped comfort the afflicted. It is the act of care itself which may have helped bring healing.

For medieval women, healing could be a double-edged sword. For example, in the *Distaff Gospels*, it was implied that one of the old women proclaiming their 'gospels', Berthe du Corne, practiced medicine (formal medicine) without permission, having learned the trade from her physician father. This idea is used to comic effect, and there is the air of something unseemly about her medical knowledge; this may have actually been true in general as medicine became more professionalized. Women who were not commonly permitted to practice academic or theoretical medicine had to be careful about garnering the attention of local authorities. There is the famous case in France of Peretta Perone, who claimed to be a physician and was in fact prosecuted for practicing medicine in 1410 (Dumas 1996). In addition, women who knew a good deal of herblore needed to take care that their work was seen as positive, and not in competition with physicians. There was also the possibility that a woman who was knowledgeable about medicine might be regarded suspiciously or accused of witchcraft, though this was more likely to occur in the early modern period than during the Middle Ages. However, this assumption, that women who acted as healers or midwives were regular targets of suspicions of witchcraft, has also been argued against by David Harley[2] (1990).

It is fair to say that women did serve as healers in the Middle Ages, although they were often restricted to the informal healing or midwifery that did not compete directly with physicians or surgeons. Their learning came from outside the written tradition, though elements of it may certainly have made it into the oral lore. Serving as the first line of care in the family, women have always acted as healers, even if (at least in medieval Europe) they were not allocated true positions of authority.

2 'Those who dabbled in medicine were occasionally accused but midwives were generally immune from witchcraft prosecution unless they fell foul of a zealous magistrate or there was some special local belief' (Harley 1990, p. 1).

Women as food producers

Women are the source of our first nourishment. From that point forward, they are most likely to be involved in providing us with food. Whether women grow the vegetables or tend to the animals that will serve as our food, shop for or sell edible goods, or cook food at home, women are most likely to be the ones who provide us with things to eat. While men may be more renowned as chefs or may do the heaviest agricultural labour, our everyday fare usually passes through the hands of women (DeVault 1991).

Evidence suggests that women were the primary food providers in the Middle Ages. They kept kitchen gardens, prepared food in the home, passed on their cooking implements to their daughters, churned butter, tended chickens, milked cows, brewed ale in places where that was the primary beverage, made dough to be baked in a communal oven, and kept their families fed. While the division of women's labour in food preparation was class-based, it is true that the great majority of women were involved in food preparation to a greater or lesser degree (McIntosh and Zey 1989).

There are a variety of ways to examine the role of women in the provisioning and preparation of food, but given their limitations they do not provide us with a full accounting of women's efforts. One source is the pictorial record:

> As we see again and again in the pictorial record, close by the fireplace – where busy hands would be skimming the broth, stirring the frumenty with the big wooden spoon that was the special symbol of a cook, or basting the roast with the juices that fell into the dripping pan – a broyeur, or the cook herself, would, with great exertion, be pounding a pestle in a big mortar set on the table or even on the floor (Redon, Sabban, and Serventi 1998 [1991], 16).

The association of women with food provision was so strong that in the Bamburg witch trials of the Early Modern period (1626-1631), women were associated with poisoning, the ultimate betrayal of their roles as nurturers and food providers. Women were accused of stealing milk, of poisoning food, and of other potential crimes within the realm of their daily duties.

> Food preparation was generally the province of women, but so too were market-gardening and butter making, two of [a woman accused of witchcraft's] main sources of income. Note here, though, that it is specifically the economic activities – production of food for market – that are gendered, not the practice of witchcraft (Smith 2007b, 110-111).

There are other examples of women being accused of poisoning, turning milk sour, and other misdeeds related directly to their roles as food providers. The opposite of the generous nurturing woman is the one who withholds care, is too lazy to cook or procure food, or who malevolently turns her duties as a woman on their head by providing food that can injure or kill. In Sweden, a dairy-centric culture, there were a variety of folk beliefs involving milking. Women were accused of making deals with the devil to steal milk, sometimes by the means of a constructed 'milk hare' made of sticks, wool, fingernails, or human hair with a few drops of blood. It was believed that the milk hare would be sent to drink milk from neighbours' cows, and then bring it back, vomiting it into a cask. 'It is said that a female milk stealer's powers were so great, that she could milk blood from the neighbour's cow if she did not stop in time; this could count for the death or sickness of an animal' (Salomonsson 1994). While this belief was recorded in the modern era, folklore tends to be conservative and it is possible that similar beliefs were present in the Middle Ages. For example, milk-stealing creatures appear in medieval church paintings. During the witch-craze hysteria in the seventeenth and eighteenth centuries, women were accused of stealing milk with the devil's help (Nilden-Wall and Wall 1993).

In Ireland, cows and dairying were also of major importance. An eighth-century law, *Cáin Lánamna*[3], stated that a husband could not get rid of cows without the consent of his wife, and stipulated the division of dairy products in case of divorce, favouring the women and pointing to the important female role in dairying. As was the case in Sweden, the Irish had folk beliefs about 'dairy luck', and the potential theft of milk from neighbours by means of magic. The eve of Beltane (May 1) marked a critical time in the preservation of dairy luck, and it was also the time at which cows were most susceptible to theft. On this evening and early morning, even walking across another's land and getting the dew on one's shoes could take all the dairy luck from a family, especially in the case of a woman. Women were most often accused of stealing milk, and it was thought that women had methods of collecting dew on Beltane to steal milk-luck. In a variation on the Swedish milk-hare, according to a twelfth-century manuscript by Giraldus Cambrensis, some women were capable of shape-shifting and might turn themselves into milk-stealing hares (Lysaght 1994).

There is a variety of evidence that suggests women were the primary cooks and had a basic education in preparing food, learned by watching their mothers and being given increasingly complicated food preparation

3 *The Law of Couples.*

duties as they matured. As part of an oral tradition, however, this was not well-documented (Redon, Sabban, and Serventi 1998 [1991]). One particularly striking written example is contained in the *Viandier*, attributed to the French chef Taillevent. In a later edition of this work (anonymously edited), under the heading 'Lesser Pottages', we find the comment: 'women are masters of these and each one knows how to make them[4]. These lesser pottages were described as uncomplicated dishes, made out of beans, peas, and pork offal, the common foods of lesser tables. In households not possessing the means to hire professional cooks (i.e. most of them), women would have been the primary cooks (Tomasik 2007, 201, fn).

One way for women to earn money was to go to market, selling extra eggs, garden produce, ale, and other products of the house and kitchen gardens (Hanawalt 1986). This type of commerce was small in scale, and conducted primarily by women. There are various accounts of women in villages and towns selling fruit or vegetables in the street, while male traders tended to deal in meat and more specialized goods (Dyer 2009). For example, in areas where milk products were consumed, women did most of the dairying, and produced their own butter and cheese, sometimes selling the excess informally. When we find more substantial trade in dairy products, men – such as cheese-mongers, who sold a larger quantity and variety of cheeses – would be the ones selling (Woolgar 2009b). In France, men were in charge of the spice trade, made specialized sauces for purchase, professionally roasted and carved geese, or made and sold oublies[5] (Redon, Sabban, and Serventi 1998 [1991], 17).

Women occasionally participated in larger-scale agriculture, in addition to tending the kitchen garden, which helped to supplement the daily meals. During the harvest, for example, scenes of daily life, such as those from the *Très Riches Heures du Duc de Berry*, show women helping with the harvest of grains. This was not uncommon in medieval depictions of the 'Labours of the Year'. While actual scenes of cooking in these images is relatively rare, both women and men are shown in activities that typify food provision or eating (Henisch 1995). Women and children were also given the right to 'glean', or to pick up grains that were dislodged during the harvest, and had fallen to the ground. In some cases, women could engage in highly paid irregular work when there was a shortage of men to take the jobs or landlords had taken an active interest in planting more crops. Women participating in the labour force may be, for example, one of the factors that reduced the age of

4 'femmes en sont maitresses et chascun le sçait faire'

5 Thin wafer waffles.

marriage and increased the number of children born in the third quarter of the fourteenth century (Woolgar 2009a).

Women could also be associated with food in medieval hagiography. Two works in the 1980s explored the concept of 'holy anorexia', or women's refusal of food as evidence of saintliness in hagiography, analysing it as a way for women to gain power that they might not otherwise have: *Holy Anorexia* by Rudolph Bell (1985) and *Holy Feast, Holy Fast* by Carol Walker Bynum (1987). One example of the link between saintliness, food, and nurturing comes from the life of Catherine of Siena. In one story, St. Catherine is able to multiply loaves of bread, much as Jesus did with the miraculous aid of the Virgin Mary: 'The kitchen was women's work, and who was more domestic and maternal that the mother of Jesus herself?' (Vitale 2010). In another hagiographic example, the nun Radegund miraculously had a cask of wine at her monastery that never ran dry. While Radegund herself often fasted to the extreme, she was known for providing meals for the poor, saving them from starvation (Effros 2002).

In fabliaux, women were beaten for not cooking for the household, men were teased for being subservient to their wives, cunning women plied their lovers with food while hiding the fact from their husbands, and gluttony and food imagery abounded. Seeing women preparing food in the fabliaux is important, as we actually don't have much textual evidence for what seems to have been common expectation, that women cook for their families. In fact, in the fabliaux, women failing to provide meals for their husbands are a source of comedy (and derision). In one of the more violent fabliaux, 'Master Ham and Naggie, His Wife', a nagging wife spoils her husband's food on purpose, because she hates him and controverts all his wishes. She feeds him peas rather than the greens he requested, or greens rather than peas, taking care to ruin them. When he requests boiled beef, she drops the cooked meat in the ashes.

In the end, Master Ham has enough and the two of them literally have a knock-down, drag-out fight for his pants – whoever wins and wears them will be in charge. Naggie loses, Master Ham puts on the pants, and Naggie must promise in front of the neighbours to obey her husband. A good wife, by contrast, makes sure her family is fed well, and domestic harmony ensues, as with the peasant wife in 'Constant du Hamel'[6]:

> ... Constant du Hamel,
> who of all this was ignorant,
> and to his wife, who simply went
> back home as quickly as she could

6 All quotes are from the translations by Dubin 2013.

and give her workingman his food
and sent him to his daily toil
of planting crops and tilling soil (lines 138-144).

Nurturing and gender

Women, as wives and mothers, were expected to be a nurturing presence in the family. They breastfed babies, cared for and fed young children, cooked for their families, tended the household garden and domestic animals, cared for sick family members by providing comfort and nursing, and perhaps with folk knowledge of how to recognize and treat common symptoms. Women, as we have seen, who did not fit into this idealized role were the objects of laughter and derision or, as was the case with some ecclesiastical writers, taken to task for not fulfilling God's appointed role for them.

It has been increasingly recognized that the domestic space is not well-documented, and thus the labours of women are often obscured (Gilchrist 2012). While there has been significant progress in recent years in trying to understand the domestic space and the life lived within it, it wasn't something that medieval people wrote much about, aside from general instructions on family life, religious instruction on the roles of men and women in the family, and various didactic literature outlining the duties of women in the household and towards the family. It wasn't until the late Middle Ages and Early Modern period that we begin to see literature specifically aimed at teaching women how to cook and care for the household, such as the *Ménagier de Paris* (Greco and Rose 2009), or the later *English Huswife* by Gervaise Markham (Markham 1986 [1615]). These sources, while informative, tell us more about the ideals to which the bourgeoisie aspired than the actualities of everyday life. Fabliaux give us a glimpse into daily life (Gordon 2007), but depicting domestic life was not their particular aim.

Archaeology provides us with more concrete evidence of the domestic space and its uses (Greenville 2000; Gilchrist 2012), as well as abundant evidence of how households were laid out, what implements were used to aid in daily tasks, how many generations lived under one roof, and so on; however, we must be cautious about interpreting any single area as gendered space (Gilchrist 1999). Only the well-to-do had separate kitchens, and for most people the entire household was used at various times by all members of the family. We know or have inferred a great deal about what was cooked, how it was cooked, where provisions came from, how the religious calendar affected the choice of food available, where food was stored, and how people dealt with food shortages.

What is more difficult to divine are the specific roles women played in the household. As mentioned previously, the written record is somewhat lacking in the details of everyday life. This is where anthropological approaches may help us infer the roles played by women as nurturers and healers.

> These historical narratives contradict anthropological approaches that highlight the contributions of women to a great diversity of historically specific systems of organizing health care. And they also contravene what we know of medieval people's perceptions – implicit and explicit – of the importance of women in attending health (Cabré 2008, 23).

While cultures do, of course, vary, for the majority of the world women have served in the role of primary caretaker of young children, and as the primary source of food and cooking for the family. They are also, as noted above, the first to treat illness, and to provide nursing care for those with extended illness. This is not to say, of course, that men don't play a role in these things, but the burden of both fell primarily to women.

What feeding and healing both have in common is care for the body. Women are the only ones who can grow a new being. As part of her own body, she is already the caretaker, though that care may be more or less intentional. We know from the historical record that women and society placed great emphasis on having children (Toulalan 2014; Fissell 2004). In the medieval era, the exception to this would be, of course, nuns or the infertile. But pregnancy was the common experience for the majority of women. The intimate act of carrying a child starts the role of woman as caretaker. After the birth of a child, itself a momentous act, the new mother was the primary caretaker of the infant unless the family was wealthy enough to hire a wet-nurse or a nursemaid. We know that mothers prayed for and desired healthy children and successful pregnancies. Towards that end, mothers breastfed their children (or made sure they were breastfed) and were the first to introduce solid foods[7]. Mothers were and are highly attuned to the needs of their children, and also to the signs that they might be ill.

Today, in countries with good sanitation and access to medical care, most routine childhood illnesses are not life-threatening. The threat was greater in the Middle Ages. A mother would have been taught how to prepare foods suitable for an invalid or a young child, how to care for a feverish child, how to make a congested child breathe easier, and when to determine if a child

7 When looking at cultures around the world, the first solid foods could consist of gruel or other soft-cooked grain, or could have been firmer food chewed first by the mother.

needed more help than the mother could give. A wise woman, medicus, apothecary, or physician could be consulted in more grave situations, if the family had the means to do so. But even if a physician could be consulted, the doctor is only there for a relatively short while. The nursing care falls to the family, and most especially the mother. Women care for our bodies when we are young, and tend to our illnesses even when we are older.

Pushed out of the medical profession, pushed out of the kitchen

As guilds and the professionalization of food preparation pushed women out of brewing (Bennett 1996) and limited their access to provisioning businesses, so the increasing professionalization of medicine and the demand for university-trained physicians eclipsed women's roles as healers.

The role of women in the medical field is well documented, although accounts vary as to what the available evidence suggests about why women were increasingly excluded from the professional medical field. For example, some authors have noted that the men took over the treatment of women at the expense of more informally trained midwives – women who supported other women in pregnancy and childbirth – while others have suggested that women's decreased role was the result of increased demand for physicians and male-midwives (King 2007). While some of that work was completed after the medieval period, women became legally excluded from medical education and the practice of physicians. While women continued to serve as midwives, there was a concerted effort on the part of the medical field to denigrate the work of midwives and to exclude them from the birth process (Harris-Stoertz 2014). Professional female midwives, apart from lay-midwives, did continue to exist and were less excluded from the medical field (Piper 2010).

It is also true that we can trace the development of professional chefs and the exclusion of women from that category as well. In the medieval period, as far as we can tell, most women were involved in the everyday production of food for the family. For the majority of women belonging to the peasant class, that meant preparing stews and soups, purchasing bread, making dough to be baked by the local baker, and sometimes milling if no miller were available or if flour were prohibitively expensive[8]. As mentioned above,

8 Typically, a miller would charge a certain percentage of the grain to produce flour from grains grown by a family. Likewise, the baker would sell ready-made loaves, but would also bake loaves of dough made by the woman of the household, again charging a percentage of the dough for this service, dough that would be baked and sold.

peasant women typically kept household gardens (as opposed to the tilled fields of the family or community, worked mainly by men, but also by women during harvest time), and could draw on those for vegetables or fruit in season. Chickens would be kept for eggs, and possibly a cow or two for milk. Meat was eaten, but far less often than by the upper classes, usually added as flavouring for a stew or pottage rather than a roast, except for special occasions. Families might slaughter and preserve a pig or two for meat, but beef was also fairly common (Woolgar, Serjeantson, and Waldron 2009).

The activities of peasant women were not considered important enough (or at least exceptional enough) to record in any detail, so we have indirect evidence for women's activities. Some of the evidence for women's culinary activities can be found in illustrations, in stories about women who refuse to do their duty by cooking, in representations in misericords, in wills that passed down cooking implements from mother to daughter, in didactic literature, in religious literature emphasizing the duties of wives and mothers, to some extent in the archaeological evidence (although that is sometimes harder to identify by gender), and so on. That women had a duty to prepare meals for their families was so taken for granted, that we find only indirect evidence for it. Recipe books written by and for women would not begin to appear until the 1600s (Cabanillas 2017), as more women became literate and sought books of household cookery.

In some areas, women were also in charge of preparing or helping to prepare beverages. Women in England, for example, regularly brewed ale, a mildly alcoholic drink that could be made with common household items, such as a cauldron. It was not preserved and bottled, however, so it needed to be brewed every few days. It was the primary household drink for both peasant farmers and town dwellers until beer, preserved with hops, became more common in the late fourteenth and early fifteenth centuries. The brewing of beer required a more complicated process and specialized equipment, and came to be brewed primarily by men (Bennett 1996).

This is by way of contrast with relatively well-to-do families. If we take, for example, *Le Ménagier de Paris*, a manuscript from the very late fourteenth century, we see a guidebook for the proper behaviour of a wife written by her much older husband, ostensibly to help educate her in her proper duties. Aside from the fact that some of the lessons he teaches are a bit heavy-handed in terms of duty and obedience[9], the manuscript does also

9 Take, for example, the story of Griselda, which seems to have circulated in the later medieval period. Griselda, a beautiful young woman from common origins, marries a king. Although she seems to be kind, attentive, and obedient to a fault, the king decides to test her. Through a series

contain a number of recipes for the edification of a new wife. The recipes here, judging by the ingredients used and the time and techniques involved in preparation, are to be made to impress. As a bourgeois woman, the author's wife would have been expected to be familiar enough with food preparation that she could do some cooking herself, as well as direct a female servant or servants in food preparation. The recipes are likely derived from some early recipe collections written by royal cooks (Greco and Rose 2009). Still, the bourgeois household provides an intermediate point between the peasant and the aristocratic households. Women were familiar with cooking, but were also partners in the upwardly mobile aspirations of their husbands, and this meant cooking to impress – either cooking herself in less wealthy households, or directing (female) servants in wealthier homes.

In the aristocratic household, the kitchen was the domain of men. Cooking for the palace or manor house was hot, gruelling work with blasting fires, knives, and massive quantities of food and intricate preparations; a chef ruled the kitchen, although the menu may have been dictated by the head of the family or his agent. Illustrations of kitchens typically show tough-looking men doing the hard work, while boys turned spits for roasting. Women are never depicted as being present, as they are in peasant or sometimes bourgeois households. It was from these kitchens that the first recipe collections begin to appear. Feasts prepared in these kitchens could be lavish, with fifty or more different dishes prepared for a feast. The daily diet might be shaped by the advice of a physician, but a feast was a time to show off power and wealth, and elaborate and expensive dishes were expected in quantity.

After the medieval period, men remained in charge of aristocratic kitchens. While in cities women might be involved in the preparation of street food or informal fare alongside the men, the prestigious food was made by men. Women might try to stretch their abilities through the preparation of some fancier dishes, but the earliest cookbooks were not written for them: they were written for other male professional chefs. In France, as a result of the French Revolution – which turned the aristocratic world on its head – chefs who had cooked for aristocrats began to bring fine dining to the cities through a recreation of their kitchens, but this time selling

of events, which involve leading her to believe he has sent their children away to be killed, to sending her away, to making her help prepare a feast for his 'new wife' (actually their grown daughter), she remains pleasant and obedient throughout. At the end, all is revealed, Griselda is united with her children and her husband, and all praise her kindness and obedience. The author of the manuscript tells his new wife he doesn't expect her devotion to be that sorely tested, but that, you know, obedience is a good thing.

food to those who could pay for it. The precursors of the modern French restaurant kitchens, run almost military style, these kitchens also remained almost exclusively male until relatively recently. Just as with medicine, the professional kitchen was run by men, with professionals trained by other men (Parkhurst-Ferguson 2004).

In fact, the professionalisation of both cooking and medicine proceeded along similar lines. Where guilds were instituted, women were only a small minority of the membership, if admitted at all. Where university degrees are concerned, the more established the university became, and the more medicine became professionalised, the fewer women were trained and recognized as professionals. Still, women continued to cook in the homes of the humble and provide basic medical care for their families through knowledge of folk medicine.

In the next few chapters, we will examine medieval theories of medicine and health more closely, looking primarily at the written tradition, but suggesting areas where evidence for traditional and/or folk medicine might be uncovered. In tracing the written medical tradition and its relationship to food and diet linked to women's health, we'll focus on texts that feature gynaecology and obstetrics, as this is where the medical literature addresses women directly.

2 Medieval Theories of Nutrition and Health

Abstract

Ancient Greek humoral theory, as formulated primarily by Hippocrates and Galen, formed the basis of theoretical medicine in the Middle Ages. This chapter provides a brief overview of humoral theory, and explains how diet was directly related to disease and health in the Greek medical system. This chapter also traces some of the changes and modifications of humoral theory which took place through the Middle Ages.

Keywords: Hippocrates, Galen, humoral theory, non-naturals, natural philosophy, Arabic Systematists

Our understanding of food and health is, arguably, primarily culture-based. Most cultures develop their own ideas about the relationship between food and health. While today we like to think the study of food and its effects on our health is based purely on science, a good argument can be made that it is not (Chen 2008). This is not to ignore or deny the work done in nutrition science, but even that science is culture-bound. What is considered proper and healthy to eat can be based simply on social custom or folk medicine, or it can be attached to a grand theory of the functioning of the body and the role of food in the maintenance of health. The food of India, for example, is understood within the Ayurvedic system. Another comprehensive health tradition is related to Chinese medicine and its influence on Chinese cuisine. Every culture has its ideas of what is healthy and unhealthy, complete with explanations. Also, traditional ideas of illness and health embedded in folk remedies remain strong over many generations, even when existing alongside professionalized medicine (Hand 1976, 2). There is no reason to assume this was not also the case in medieval Europe, where, no doubt, folk medicine existed side by side with (and perhaps sometimes was indistinguishable from) professional theoretical medicine. While some historians deny the

Vaughan, Theresa A., *Women, Food, and Diet in the Middle Ages: Balancing the Humours.* Taylor & Francis Group, 2020
DOI: 10.5117/9789462989382_CH02

existence of a 'popular medicine', or posit that what we refer to as popular medicine was simply a bastardized version of theoretical medicine, others take the opposite view (Gentilcore 2004). Folklorists and anthropologists know that theories of medicine (and the role of food within folk medicine) are pervasive, sometimes borrowing from a written tradition, but also influencing that tradition.

In medieval Europe food traditions varied from place to place and, perhaps more strikingly, from one social class to another. An understanding of what was healthy to eat among the literate was based on Greek natural philosophy and the development of medicine. The Greek system of understanding diet and health spread throughout the Mediterranean world and beyond through the writings of natural philosophers and physicians, most notably Hippocrates and Galen. This philosophical and medical tradition, having taken root in the Roman Empire, spread into the Byzantine. It was borrowed by the great Arab and Jewish philosophers and systematists, influencing the Muslim world, where, organized and expanded, it eventually made its way back to Western Europe via the great Muslim civilizations and Byzantium. At this stage, the Greek system also absorbed learning that remained from before the fall of the Western Roman Empire, preserved largely in monasteries.

The goal of this chapter is to explain some of the basics of this cultural system by looking at works from Hippocrates and Galen, explaining the fundamentals of humoral theory, and briefly outlining some of the major works on diet and health throughout the Middle Ages. It bears keeping in mind that we are tracing here the formal tradition of the literate. To what extent these theories influenced the common people in Classical Greece and Rome, and illiterate medieval people, remains to be seen. It is harder to grasp and understand folk theories of health and medicine, or even how medicine was actually practiced by trained physicians.

The Greek tradition

Theoretical medicine in the Middle Ages was derived from writings of the Greco-Roman world. The Greeks based their understanding of the proper functioning of the body on the existence of four 'humours', each with its own associated substance. The humours circulated through the body, and a healthy body must be balanced. An overabundance of one humour could cause illness. The balance of the four humours was greatly affected, it was thought, by the foods that one consumed. Thus, from the

Greco-Roman period, theoretical medicine placed great importance on the diet as fundamental for the maintenance of good health and treatment of disease.

The work of a number of Greek philosophers forms the basis of humoral theory. The earliest of these philosophers, the Pre-Socratics, sought to understand the nature of matter – what made up the stuff of life. Each speculated about what made up the world, based on philosophical reasoning. The Pre-Socratics played a role in determining which elements were primary in terms of the composition of matter, and therefore eventually of the humours. Humoral theory contains elements of the thinking of Anaximenes (c. 586-c. 526 BCE, Miletus), Heraclitus (c. 535-c. 475 BCE, Ephesus, Persia), and Thales (c. 624-c. 546 BCE, Miletus). For Anaximenes, air was the source of all things; for Heraclitus, the primary element was fire. According to Thales, everything was made of water. These simplistic statements are far more nuanced in the written record, but as Greek philosophy grew and expanded, the ideas for fundamental parts of nature emerged. From these three Pre-Socratic monists, we get three of the four primary elements that make up humoral theory.

Other early philosophers contributed to the formation of the basics of humoral theory. For example, Empedocles (495-435 BCE, Sicily) believed that four primary elements make up the world – earth, air, fire, and water. Zeno (495-425 BCE, Velia, Italy) introduced the idea that everything has the qualities of heat or coldness, moistness or dryness. This would be fundamental to the theory of humoral complexion and its implications. Of these philosophers, the most influential on Hippocrates would be Empedocles. Elements of the theory of humours preceded Hippocrates: '(1) a medical tradition that regarded the humours as a cause of illness, (2) principles of Pythagorean philosophy concerning harmony, balance, and tetrads, (3) Empedocles' theory of the primary elements of the universe, (4) the doctrine of qualities that evolved when the theory of elements was applied to mankind' (Stelmack and Stalikos 1991, 256).

Hippocrates (460-370 BCE, Kos, Greece) and the writers of the Hippocratic Corpus – one of the two chief theoretical views of bodily functioning which influenced medieval medicine – the other being derived from Aristotle – were the first to connect the four qualities of Zeno with the four elements of Empedocles. The prototype of humoral theory first appears in the Hippocratic text *On the Nature of Man*[1] in about 400 BCE. In its estimation, the four qualities are connected with four major types of bodily fluids

1 Generally attributed to Polybus.

(Adamson 1995, 11). Within the body, the four humours or bodily fluids were phlegm, black bile, yellow bile, and blood. Each was connected to one of the four primary substances: earth, air, fire and water. Blood, warm and moist, was associated with the qualities of air; yellow bile, warm and dry, was associated with the fire; black bile, cold and dry, was connected with the qualities of earth; and phlegm, cold and moist, took on the qualities of water (Stelmack and Stalikos 1991, 258).

All consumable substances were classified by their nature. Plant and animal, living and non-living things were the product of two binary oppositions: moist or dry, and cold or hot (or cooling and heating). Thus, four compositions were available: moist and cold, moist and hot, dry and cold, and dry and hot. According to Philistion of Locri (c. fourth century BCE), fire was associated with heat, air with cold, water with moistness, and earth with dryness. As outlined in *On the Nature of Man*, part of the Hippocratic Corpus, these relationships are delineated into four bodily fluids:

BLOOD: hot and wet, associated with spring
PHLEGM: cold and wet, associated with winter
BLACK BILE: cold and dry, associated with fall
YELLOW BILE: hot and dry, associated with summer

In the other works of the Hippocratic Corpus, some further associations were made:

BLOOD: heart, childhood
PHLEGM: brain/head, old age
BLACK BILE: quartan fever, adulthood (ages 25-45)
YELLOW BILE: liver, adolescence

The authors of the Hippocratic Corpus wrote widely on all areas of health. The Corpus contains commentary on women's health, but chiefly from the point of view of disorders of the uterus, which were legion. The Greeks believed the uterus could cause problems for women's health far beyond what is typically associated with uterine health today[2]. Sometimes, recommendations for

2 As discussed later in this volume, they believed the uterus could move from its usual position and wander about the abdomen, causing illness. In the medieval texts, this is referred to as 'suffocation of the uterus' and various remedies are offered to entice it back into its proper place.

diet or certain tastes are included in the description of female diseases. In *Diseases of Women 1*, for example, causes and complications involved with restriction of the menstrual flow is examined, a concern that would be addressed by medieval medical authors.

The dietary recommendations of the Hippocratic Corpus would form the basis of dietary recommendations for health in the written Greco-Roman tradition, and on into the Middle Ages and beyond. Here, we can see the prescription for food with a certain quality – dryness – meant to counteract the abundant moisture of the phlegm. In addition, to counteract the inflated belly, the woman should not overindulge in food and wine, which would aggravate the condition, particularly in 'fleshy' women. These recommendations are based upon humoral theory as it had developed to this point.

Aristotle (384-322 BCE, Stagira, Greece) also addressed some of these subjects. He emphasized that opposites cannot occur together; things could be hot and dry, or hot and wet, or cold and dry, or cold and wet. You could not have substances or living things be both hot and cold, or both wet and dry. He also introduced the idea of the four temperaments, which were associated with the four bodily fluids. For example, a person with a preponderance of blood would have a sanguine personality; a person with a preponderance of phlegm would be phlegmatic; a preponderance of yellow bile would cause a choleric personality; and someone with a preponderance of black bile would have a melancholic personality. These ideas would go on to affect medieval dietary theories and recommendations. Aristotle also expounded upon the differences between men and women in terms of their humoral composition. He argued that female bodies were colder, and the formation of the seed which could produce an embryo necessitated abundant heat (so that the material could be fully cooked, and whole). This had implications for his ideas of the generation of the embryo: women being cold-natured, they could not fully cook their own seed, so the uterus would provide only a place for the housing of the embryo, while the male seed was the generative principle (York 2012, 62). The theory that the male provided a viable seed while women provided a place for that seed to grow, would influence certain schools of natural philosophy and later the outlook of the Church, but was not the dominant interpretation found in the Middle Ages.

Later medical writers, such as Soranus of Ephesus (first to second century CE), would add detail to Aristotle's theory of personality traits. While Aristotle concentrated primarily on melancholic personalities, Soranus first gave detailed descriptions of all four temperaments. He also related the bodily fluids to character traits. Soranus features further in Chapter Three as a noted writer on gynaecological and obstetric medicine. Although his work was influential at the time of his writing, it was largely eclipsed by the work of Galen, and therefore had relatively little influence on the medical traditions of Western Europe. The Pneumatic School[3] added time of day, week of the month, two fevers, and male and female to the basic divisions listed above (Adamson 1995, 13).

Galen of Pergamum

Galen (130-210 CE, Pergamum), who lived during the Roman Empire and wrote in the Greek of the Hellenistic world, had the most direct influence on medieval medicine. He was trained in medicine in Smyrna, Corinth, and Alexandria. Although some schools were based around various philosophical positions, there was no set medical curriculum (Grant 2000, 2). Well-versed himself in the Greek philosophical tradition, Galen combined Plato, Aristotle, and the Pneumatic School with the theories of the Hippocratic Corpus, particularly from *On the Nature of Man*. His work, and the body of literature which sprang from it, was the most frequently used in Europe of the Middle Ages (Adamson 1995). His fame was such that in CE 169, he was invited by Marcus Aurelius to become physician to the royal family, and he spent the rest of his life in Rome (Grant 2000, 2). While the work of Aristotle was also influential in the realm of natural philosophy and occasionally medicine, Galen was the touchstone for theoretical medicine and its practice, combined with traditional medical knowledge. It is theoretical medicine, however, which we can trace through the extant literature.

Among the additions Galen made to the ideas of the Hippocratic Corpus were the four qualities of taste: sweet, sour/spicy, bitter, and salty. He connected each of these fundamental types of taste to the four bodily fluids. Blood paired with sweet, phlegm with salty, black bile with sour, and yellow bile with bitter. He also clearly correlated the four elements (earth, air, fire, water) with the four qualities (hot, dry, cold, wet) and the four fluids (blood, phlegm, black bile, yellow bile). As these groupings of characteristics developed, Galen furthered the classification of the body and its qualities with anatomy, age, diet, and disease. By linking together numerous factors, the body, its functioning, and its influences could be addressed in a logical

3 The Pneumatic school, based upon the ideas of Plato and Aristotle, relied upon the principle that *pneuma*, or spirit, was the primary foundation of living things, rather than the atoms of the Methodic School of medicine.

manner, with connections and linkages making sense of the baffling array of diseases, temperaments, and body types.

Galen developed the idea of temperaments based upon his classifications. Differing temperaments could be explained by the varying qualities and their balance in each person. He proposed nine temperaments (adding to the four outlined by Soranus). Four temperaments were based upon a prevalence of one quality prevailing, four based upon the balance of two qualities, and one with perfect balance of qualities. The four least desirable temperaments were those in which only one bodily fluid was dominant. The most desirable temperament was one in which all four humours were in balance. In Galen's treatise *On the Natural Faculties*, the term 'temperament' relates directly to the four qualities: hot, cold, moist, dry. These were the four qualities that could be assigned to everything in nature, and would ultimately influence the dietary recommendations of theoretical medicine throughout the Middle Ages. In addition, the designation of the four humours and their resulting temperaments did not refer only to mood or character. The humours, their balance and their excesses, were the determinants of physical shape, constitution, and the basis of illness.

In an extended list of correlations listed in Hippocrates' *Nature of Man*, Galen added the following, noted in bold face (Adamson 1995, 14):

Figure 2.1 Four humours and their characteristics after Galen

BLOOD	PHLEGM
hot and wet	cold and wet
Spring	Winter
heart	brain
childhood	old age
air	**water**
red	**white**
sweet	**salty**
	female principle
continuous fever	**quotidian fever**
BLACK BILE	YELLOW BILE
cold and dry	hot and dry
Autumn	Summer
adulthood	liver
quartan fever	adolescence
earth	**fire**
black	**yellow**
sour	**bitter**
	male principle
spleen	**tertian fever**

Despite this growing list, Galen wrote neither abundantly nor systematically on the temperaments. A melancholic personality and its relationship to black bile had long been noted, including by Hippocrates. Galen did introduce other elements, but later medieval writers would expound upon them.

Medieval writers made a number of additions. The four temperaments were given names – sanguine, phlegmatic, melancholic, and choleric – based upon the humour in excess.

Figure 2.2 Four humours and personality types

Greek Term	English Translation	Personality Type
Sanguis	Blood	Sanguine
Flegma	phlegm	Phlegmatic
Cole	yellow bile	Choleric
melas cole	black bile	melancholic

While the names for the substances of the humours existed even before Hippocrates, it was not until the twelfth century that the characteristic personality types got their names (Stelmack and Stalikos 1991, 257).

Beyond adding the names of the four temperaments, medieval writers also added the four cardinal directions, the four evangelists (not Matthew, Mark, Luke and John, but, idiosyncratically, Mark, John, Peter, and Paul), and four of the modes of ancient music. And so, we end up with the following correspondences (Adamson 1995, p. 15):

Figure 2.3 Medieval four humours and their characteristics

BLOOD	PHLEGM
hot and wet	cold and wet
Gemini, Taurus, Aries	Pisces, Aquarius, Capricorn
Lydian Mode	Dorian Mode
Jupiter	Moon
Apostle Mark	Apostle Peter
sanguine	phlegmatic
serene	idle
unruffled	foolish
morning	evening
continuous fever	quotidian fever
red	white
sweet	salty
air	water
childhood	old age
Spring	winter

BLACK BILE	YELLOW BILE
cold and dry	hot and dry
Libra, Scorpio, Sagittarius	Virgo, Leo, Cancer
Mixo-Lydian Mode	Phrygian Mode
Saturn	Mars
Apostle John	Apostle Paul
melancholic	choleric
stubborn	bold
insolent	exuberant
afternoon	noon
quartan fever	tertian fever
black	yellow
sharp/sour	bitter
earth	fire
adulthood	youth
Autumn	Summer

Medieval writers, feeling the need to systematize a number of areas of study and inquiry, aligned and categorized seemingly non-medical or anatomical traits with the four humours. Many of these additions remained in the realm of natural philosophy and theology, rather than making an impact on theoretical medicine. They are, however, ways of organizing knowledge into a systematic whole.

Galen wrote about the various qualities of foods and their usefulness in maintaining health and in the treatment of disease. His works specifically on diet include: *On Black Bile*, *On Uneven Bad Temperament*, *On the Causes of Disease*, *On Barley Soup*, and the three books of *On the Powers of Foods* (Grant 2000). However, he did not mention the humoral system directly when writing about food. Galen also added levels of intensity to his system.

> Like Hippocrates, Galen distinguishes between pharmacopoeia which is capable of altering the *physis*[4], and foodstuffs which merely increase the substance of the body. Since a number of foodstuffs can also alter the *physis*, the distinction between foodstuffs and drugs becomes blurred, which may account for the inclusion of various items in both categories (Adamson 1995, 16).

The balance of humours within a person's body gave each person a unique complexion. Complexion here does not necessarily have to do with the quality of the skin, although some, such as Hildegard of Bingen (1098-1179

4 *Physis* is usually translated as 'nature' or 'natural', here the natural body, as opposed to *nomos*, or things that come about by convention.

CE), felt the general health of an individual could be determined through an examination of the face or skin. Rather, complexion refers to individual humoral composition. While complexion is related to the notion of temperaments, they are not the same thing. Temperament was originally conceived of as stemming from the balance of the four qualities of hot, cold, moist, and dry. Complexion, instead, was based upon the balance of the bodily fluids known as humours – related to the four qualities, as explained above – and the humour found in excess.

The idea that what one consumed could alter or affect individual complexion developed early on. According to Aristotle, the nutritive, or vegetative aspects of the spirit/soul controlled the areas of nutrition, growth, and reproduction. The digestive organs were responsible for breaking down food into useable components. The liver was the primary organ involved in digestion, and blood, composed of humoral blood plus an admixture of the other humours, was carried from the digestive organs to the rest of the body (Siraisi 2009, 108).

Complexion and the effect of foodstuffs on complexion was also deeply embedded in the Hippocratic tradition. The dietary rules laid out by the ancient Greeks formed the basis of medieval writing on diet. The rules of diet were based upon the idea that disease and general health were a matter of humoral balance or imbalance. Imbalances were responsible for certain medical conditions. Various actions could affect humoral balance: ingesting prepared medications, application of heat or cold, fumigations, baths, or the consumption of a proper diet. Diet was often used in conjunction with medicine and other healing techniques in order to improve health.

According to Galen, food was chewed and entered the stomach. In the stomach the process of concoction took place (while we think of food as being digested, the Galenic tradition thought of food as being 'cooked', or concocted). Concoction requires heat, just as cooking does. Beginning in the stomach, concocted food turned into chyle, a substance that could be used by the body. Food that was not concocted became waste, which could be eliminated as faeces or other bodily wastes. The chyle itself could be diverted to the spleen, where it was turned into bile, which would return to the stomach to help the process of concoction. Other chyle was diverted to the liver, where it was further cooked. Waste from the liver was eliminated as urine. The cooked chyle would be turned into blood. Blood was sent to the right ventricle of the heart, where it would either be diverted to the lungs, or diffused through the septum to the left ventricle. In the left ventricle, the blood would be mixed with pneuma, a vital spirit from the lungs. From there it was sent to the arteries. Some would be diverted to the tissues and organs, while some was further concocted to produce warmth and energy. The waste from this last round of concoction would leave the body as sweat (Berger 1999, 17).

Also stemming from the works of Galen were two categories of things that affected health, known in English as the 'naturals' and 'non-naturals'. The naturals were physiological factors which included elements, qualities, humours, parts of the body, faculties, spirits, and temperaments. The non-naturals were lifestyle-dependent factors that included air, food and drink, evacuation and repletion, sleeping and waking, rest and motion, and passions of the mind (Jarcho 1970). 'The immediate causes of most forms of disease were attributed to shifts in the patient's complexional balance. These changes might in turn be set off by harmful changes in the non-naturals, especially food, drink, air and water' (Siraisi 2009, 123).

It follows that if a disease process could be set off by harmful changes in the non-naturals, a modification in the non-naturals (including food and drink) might stop or ameliorate the disease process. 'That a good diet ensured health was a fundamental concept of ancient medicine, since food could cause disease or restore health through its effect on the balance of the humours. Thus prevention was in every way better than a cure' (Grant 2000, 7). Greco-Roman physicians and philosophers had much to say about what was proper to eat, but all of them were based upon humoral theory as well as on the local diet. Knowledge of the humoral composition of foods and spices was essential for the prescription of a proper diet, based upon an individual's own humoral composition. There was not, however, universal agreement on the humoral composition of various foodstuffs.

Galen's most important work on diet is entitled *On the Properties of Foodstuffs*[5], or *On the Powers of Foods*. He wrote it when he had already become a well-known physician. It serves as a more or less practical manual for understanding proper diet. In it, Galen follows the work of several natural philosophers, but is most influenced by Hippocrates' work *On Diet* (Grant 2000, 10). While Galen seeks to systematize these earlier works, his dietary recommendations are still classified somewhat haphazardly. This, like other treatises by Galen, was polemical, and he clearly postures and disagrees with the works of earlier philosophers. This type of rhetorical posturing was a common practice of the time.

What did Galen advise people to eat? There are several treatises included in *On the Powers of Foods* that can enlighten us. In one short treatise, *On Barley Soup*, Galen explores the properties of barley, discusses cooking

5 *De alimentorum facultatibus*

methods, and explains how this simple dish can influence the humours when consumed. To begin, what are the properties of barley itself? 'As is universally acknowledged, barley is cooling and drying, but has a purgative and flatulent element. It's exterior husk, since it is like bran, is drier and more purgative. Its interior, resembling a sort of nutritious flesh, is purgative too, but less so than bran, although it has in itself a flatulent quality' (Grant 2000, 63). Galen then explores the grain of barley in more detail: how to determine what barley is wholesome to eat, the effect of moisture on the barley, and the necessity of using barley that is scrupulously clean. He then goes on to explain how to determine the best water in which to cook the grain, and how to recognize it. Galen discusses the best way to prepare the barley soup, so as to reduce or eliminate its more flatulent qualities. He argues that some of the common ways to prepare barley soup are incorrect, because they will result in a product that is not as healthful for the body, and includes a brief discussion on why barley soup, properly prepared, is suitable for the treatment of certain illnesses. For example, smooth, moist soup will not cause flatulence and can help treat acute fevers (Grant 2000, 65-66).

This is simply one example of Galen's analysis of food qualities, and how they can be used as a treatment for illness. It is important to understand that the theory of food and medicine being developed through the Hippocratic Corpus and works of Galen is derived from the philosophical underpinnings of natural philosophy. Galen and his successors had detailed explanations for the properties inherent in food and drink, and their positive or negative effects. A humoral theory of nutrition held that food in and of itself wasn't fully healthful, but the processing of that food or drink could be undertaken to maximize its beneficial qualities, and minimize the harmful. By the Middle Ages, the addition of herbs and spices and the development of cooking methods were used to modify the humoral qualities of food and drink, mitigating harmful effects and maximizing benefits. Spices and wines were thought to be particularly powerful tools for modifying underlying humoral qualities. In addition, spices could serve as purgatives, taken after meals to aid in digestion. Spices and wines could also provide the body with additional heat to concoct food: not simply to chase away bad humours, but also to incinerate them. Wine could be mixed directly with spices to enhance this effect (Vigarello 1993, 29-36).

There was no single proper way to prepare food, nor single best food to eat. The complexion of each individual could be analysed and a diet prescribed to help bring the body into balance. Galen saw a humorally-balanced body as a healthy body, with the belief that food and drink could be prepared in such a way that they would counteract humoral imbalances and treat illness and disease. There were some limits to the modification that could be accomplished through cooking and spicing, so some examples of food and drink were not recommended at all for certain conditions. Other foods, because of their gentleness and balance, were regularly recommended for the ill, the weak, or the recuperating. For Galen, as we have seen, barley soup was one such suggestion. Chicken, blancmange, eggs, and weak white wine or ale were a few of the foods commonly given to invalids during the Middle Ages. These items were considered not only humorally-balanced or neutral, but also easily digested (or concocted), since waste products not easily removed by the body would ultimately cause an excess of certain humours. Therefore, complete digestion was desired. In addition, none of these foods were highly spiced; all tended to be light or white in colour, and therefore were considered more delicate and easily digested.

Again, it should be emphasized that these ideas were not new to Galen, nor were they even new to Hippocrates. Rather, Galen addressed earlier arguments about the qualities of food and drink, added further explanation, systematized the arguments to some degree, and asserted his own analytical view. He also understood that knowledge of what foods to eat and how diet could be used to treat disease came not only from purely philosophical treatises, but that they were also found in simple (empirical) practical medicine, based on long experience with the treatment of patients[6]. Galen, as both a practicing physician and a person trained in natural philosophy, was poised to address knowledge from both sides – the theoretical and the practical. He was able to explain some of the practical medicine and why it worked by applying theoretical knowledge[7], assessing the effectiveness of the purely theoretical approach. Galen himself emphasized the importance of theoretical understanding and philosophical reasoning in the practice of medicine, as was appropriate for someone poised within the theoretical medical tradition, a much more intellectually privileged position. His understanding of the Hippocratic Corpus, as well as other contributions to Greek medicine, was extensive, and by pulling that corpus into a seemingly coherent whole, Galen laid the foundation for medical education for years to come. His influence is clearly evident throughout the Middle Ages and beyond (York 2012, 25).

6 For further discussion of my take on the distinctions between popular, folk, empirical, practical, and theoretical medicine in the Middle Ages, please see Chapter Four.

7 Even if that theoretical knowledge was, by contemporary standards, inaccurate.

Anthimus

Of course, diet was not the only method of treating bodily diseases and disorders in the Greco-Roman tradition. There was also a long tradition of pharmaceutical treatment. Medicines could be made from a variety of substances – herbs were especially important – but non-plant items[8] could also be used. Many medical texts contained information on treatment and diet for the ill, but also contained many recipes for the making of medicines[9]. The history of pharmacy is also enlightening in tracing the history of health care, gynaecology, and obstetrics from the Ancient world through the Early Modern period. While this work does not focus on medicine/pharmaceuticals per se, it briefly explores the uses of food in the making of medicine[10] as well as the use of food as medicine.

Anthimus (475-525 CE, Constantinople), a Byzantine physician exiled to the court of Theodoric the Great (r. 498-526 CE), was the author of *De observation ciborum* ('On the Observance of Food'), subtitled 'How all food should be eaten so that it may be properly digested and promote health, rather than cause stomach problems and persistent infirmity of the body'. This guide may have been written for the Frankish king Theodoric, advising him on diet. The effort was complicated by the fact that the Frankish diet did not conform to the Byzantine diet, and Anthimus had to modify his recommendations accordingly. Anthimus' work, while not as well-known as the Hippocratic or Galenic texts, did explore food specifically, in what would eventually become a literary tradition that would include herbals, cookbooks, and *Regimina sanitatis*[11]. Anthimus emphasized the importance of proper cooking as a means to render food easier to digest, somewhat unusual in this textual tradition. Food that had not been cooked properly, he said, causes 'a heaviness in the stomach and bowels' (Wallis 2010, 78). Poorly cooked food might be indigestible or result in waste fluids that might lead to vomiting and diarrhoea. This view informs some of the cooking of the Middle Ages, where, at least according to humoral theory, raw fruits and

8 Other substances used in making medicines were theriac, mercury, animal-derived substances, myrrh, and metals.

9 See, for example, theories of medication by the physician Asclepiades (Santacroce, Bottalico, and Charitos 2017).

10 See Chapters Five and Six especially.

11 There are a number of manuscripts that use the title *'Regimen sanitatis'*, which simply means 'rule of health'. The plural form used in this book is *Regimina sanitatis* referring both to books of that title and a genre of health literature based upon the six non-naturals, with an emphasis on food and drink.

vegetables should be consumed only rarely and with the greatest of caution. Anthimus asserted that those who take care to prepare food properly would not get ill and would not require other medicine.

Anthimus had to adapt dietary regulations to food or eating techniques that did not conform to what was typically considered healthful in the Byzantine diet. For example, the Franks had a habit of consuming raw bacon, so Anthimus had to find a way of advising against this habit without causing offense. He mentioned that roasting creates dry bacon, which produces bad humours and ill health. He suggested boiling bacon well instead and removing the rind, rendering it more digestible. When faced with the habit of eating raw bacon, he mentioned that it perhaps may serve as a means to expel 'stomach and gnawing worms' (Wallis 2010, 79). He also noted that raw bacon can be placed on both external and internal wounds to promote healing, and that it 'cleanses putrefaction' (Wallis 2010, 79). He suggested that raw bacon is an effective medicine, possibly in an attempt to curry favour with the Frankish king. It is a fine line between promoting proper theoretical medicine and currying favour with a king.

Medical writers in the medieval Islamic world

One cannot trace the history of dietary recommendations for health from the ancient world through the Middle Ages without some understanding of the influence of the Islamic world. There were numerous Arabic language contributions to the medical literature, many of them influenced by the works of Ancient Greece, which made their way into the Islamic world through translations from Greek into Arabic, or Greek to Syriac, then Arabic. These authors further systematized Greek medicine, and included some contributions from Islamic learning as well. As theoretical approaches were adopted from Greek medicine, the philosophical underpinnings of that medicine were retained and expanded. Philosophy would continue to underlie theoretical medicine for centuries to come. Some works veered from the purely philosophical, and among the Arabic medical texts were reference works for practicing physicians[12]. They contained observational accounts of diseases and symptoms, and were well regarded in the Islamic world, eventually in medieval Europe as well (Siraisi 2009, 12-13). Some of the most important Arab systematists were the encyclopaedists Avicenna (Ibn Sina, 980-1037 CE, Afshona, Uzbekistan), Averroës (Ibn Rushd, 1126-1198 CE,

12 For an overview, see (Majeed 2005).

Córdoba), and Rhazes (al-Razi, 854-925 CE, Ray, Iran). Regarding dietetics, there are several notable contributions by Arab authors.

In the tenth century, Hali Abbas (Ali ibn al-Abbas al-Magusi, tenth century CE, Ahvaz, Persia) summarized and systematized Galenic medical theory. Hali Abbas was born in Iran but practiced as a physician in Baghdad, where he founded a hospital. His most famous work is *The Complete Book of the Medical Art* (*Kitab Kamil al-sina'ah al-tibbiyah*), also called *The Royal Book* (*al-Kitab al-Malaki*). It consisted of a two-volume encyclopaedia that summarized and organized the work of Hippocrates, Galen, and Rhazes. It was translated into Latin as the *Liber pantegni*. It addressed diet by describing regimens for health. Health regulations were divided into four categories: 'medicine, deadly food, medicine as food, food alone"[13]. It addressed the non-naturals and their influence on health, as well as dealing with many other issues.

Hunain ibn Ishaq al Ibadi, known in the west as Johannitius (809-873 CE, Al-Hira), was a Nestorian Christian scholar from Iraq who also practiced medicine in Baghdad. His most popular work was *Questions on Medicine*, a translation of Galen. In it, he further addressed the six non-naturals (Adamson 1995). In his *Isagoge*, Johannitius categorized food into two types: good food and bad food. Good food generated good humours; bad food produced bad humours. Good food was defined as food with a balance of qualities that produced good blood. Bad food was humorally imbalanced and resulted in bad blood. He further subdivided good and bad food into heavy and light. When referring to meat, the best food for the body was balanced and of moderate size and activity. All foods generated one of the four humours, but those that produced red (yellow) bile, black bile, and phlegm in excess were not good for the body. He also categorized drink into three categories. In the first category, a drink such as water was of neutral value. In a second category were drinks that acted as food. In the third, a drink was both a drink and a medicine that could counteract disease. Examples of this type of drink were meliorate (hydromel)[14], mead, and spiced tonic. According to Johannitius, 'Food is useful because it restores the integrity of the body in its proper order. Drink is useful because it distributes food throughout the body. But that kind of drink which we call "potion" is useful because it changes the nature of the body into itself' (Wallis 2010, 145-146).

One of the most notable of the Arab systematists was Abū 'Alī al-Ḥusayn ibn 'Abd Allāh ibn Sīnā, or Avicenna as he was known in the West. Writing

13 *"medicina, mortifera portio, medicinales cibi*, and *solum cibus"*

14 At minimum, honey mixed with water. Other components could be added.

during the Islamic Golden Age, his primary work, *The Canon of Medicine* (*Kitab al-Qanun fi al-tibb*), gives a better description of the ambivalent nature of the non-naturals. In his writing, he attempted to synthesize the two sometimes differing views of Galen and Aristotle. He became a leading authority in the field of medicine in both the Arab and Christian worlds. Advocating a logical approach to symptoms and their diagnoses, he insisted that all symptoms must be carefully evaluated before a diagnosis to avoid prescribing incorrect treatments or pharmaceuticals. He advocated for the most conservative treatment that would be effective in alleviating symptoms. Copies of his work, translated into Latin, are found in numerous libraries in Western Europe (U.S. National Library of Medicine 2011).

Meanwhile, Magister Theodorus Priscianus (c. fourth-fifth century CE, Constantinople), writing in Latin and author of the fourth century *Diaeta Theodori*, included dietary recommendations in his own text. For example, 'two potions are listed which keep the body healthy, and guard the head, chest, and all intact inner organs ... Both are based on wine and honey with the addition of a number of spices, and seem to be variations on the popular spiced wine called *Ypocras*' (Adamson 1995, 29).

The medieval west

The dietary recommendations in the works of the Middle Ages derived from this tradition. Diseases were described in similar ways, and the use and preparation of pharmaceuticals was also based, at least in part, on the Greek medical tradition. Medicines were usually comprised of readily obtainable substances, although could also include much more rare and expensive ingredients, such as precious metals and gems (Vigarello 1993, 22, 28). The areas of diet and medicine overlap when herbs and plants, often used in cooking, were also used in the preparation of medicine. While we have some ways of exploring and understanding folk or popular medicine of the time period, it is not clear that folk remedies were extremely divergent from the basics of the humoral tradition. It is likely that folk medicine, passed along through oral tradition, also contained some influence from Greek medicine of the written tradition (Wallis 2010, 146).

Medicine in post-antiquity Western Europe took a more academic turn with medical literature associated with the city of Salerno, in Italy. Originally a resort city, it became the crossroads of European, Arabic, and Jewish medical learning. Salerno was the site of the first organized medical school in Europe. The Salernitan school of medicine was the beneficiary of

Greek and Arabic texts, some of which were newly translated into Latin. Salerno, however, had been colonized by Greeks, and the heritors of that colonization still spoke Greek. As a formal system of medical education developed, students were introduced to Greek and Arabic works (often in Latin translation) and the philosophical basis of theoretical medicine. Just as the Arabic systematists wove together the strands of Greek medicine into a more coherent and comprehensible whole, so the Salernitan writers combined this work with practical medical knowledge that came to be called *physica* (Wallis 2010, 129-131). This was as opposed to *medicina*, the practical art of treating disease. A number of medical writers' work survived even after Salerno was no longer an important medical centre. Bartholomaus of Salerno (1100 -1156 CE) wrote *The Practice of Medicine* (*Practica medicinae*). His dietary recommendations for medical treatment echo those of the Arab writers[15].

The *Trotula*, a collection of three texts purported to be written by a female physician of the medical school of Salerno named Dame Trota, proved to have a lasting influence on women's medicine through the Early Modern period. It was the most important work on gynaecology to emerge from the world of academic medicine, based largely on the ideas of Galen, along with the practical medicine taught at Salerno. Earlier gynaecological medicine in Salerno was based on Hippocratic and Methodist[16] sources. While Galen himself did not write extensively on gynaecology, his explanation of the humours and the particular application of humoral theory to women was adopted by the author of the *Trotula* (Wallis 2010, 185). The *Trotula* is explored more extensively in Chapter Five.

By the beginning of the thirteenth century, Salerno no longer played an important role in the development of medicine in Europe. Medical texts from Salerno, such as the *Trotula*, did have a lasting effect, however. Important medical schools would arise in Montpellier, Paris, Bologna, and Padua, as universities themselves arose and spread through Europe. These schools drew not just from local populations for their professoriate and student body, but from all over Europe. Latin, the common language of study, enabled students from disparate regions to communicate with each other and with instructors. Some were denied entry to medical schools and to the more theoretical learning that their curricula entailed. Jewish students were permitted to attend lectures at some medical schools, such as Montpellier,

15 There is, of course, an impressive list of faculty from Salerno, as well as other important books, such as the *Regimen sanitatis Salernitinum*.

16 Hippocrates and the Methodist school of thought were sometimes at odds with each other.

but were barred from earning degrees. Women, with a few rare exceptions, were generally forbidden to matriculate as university students (York 2012, 37).

By the end of the thirteenth century, an increasing number of medical texts became available in the vernacular languages of Europe, making them accessible to those who were literate in their own languages but not in Latin. This spread Greek and Arabic medical learning even farther than translations into Latin had done. In addition, there were the various versions of *Regimina sanitatis*, which focused primarily on the six non-naturals. These books, intended for an aristocratic audience, were considered particularly appropriate for aristocrats because medieval physicians believed that people of the nobility had a more refined and delicate complexion than the lower classes. This complexion was hereditary, and came into being at the moment of conception (Wells 2002, 20). These books tended to advise the consumption of high-quality foodstuffs, especially wild game, young poultry, bread made from refined white flour, and other delicacies. Those not of the aristocracy could get by with less refined, heartier food: older beef and pork, heavy, whole-grained bread, cabbage, and other cool weather crops (Woolgar, Serjeantson, and Waldron 2009).

In the next chapter, the specific dietary recommendations for women's health will be explored. Did recommendations for men and women differ? If so, why? How much was advice for women based upon gynaecological and obstetric concerns? Were these the only differences between male and female health? What were the specific recommendations for successful breastfeeding? How did recommendations for women change over time? These are a few of the questions to be explored.

3 The Special Problem of Nutrition and Women's Health

Abstract
In this chapter, we move beyond the basics of humoral theory to those recommendations specific to women's health. In particular, dietary recommendations for women's health are considered as they pertain to theoretical medicine but also as they concern religion and folk medicine. Specific concerns about women were typically found in gynaecological texts. Pregnancy was typically viewed as a condition which required special treatment, but dietary treatment was often similar to that used for any ill or recuperating person.

Keywords: gynaecology, obstetrics, humoral theory, pregnancy, *Trotula*, medieval medical texts

Beginning with the literature of the ancient Greeks, which formed the foundational theoretical and practical underpinnings of Western medicine, women were viewed as being physiologically related to men, but different enough to merit some separate analysis of their bodies, digestion, and reproductive function. In fact, a number of Greek writers on natural philosophy and medicine considered them essentially to be defective men – not quite fully formed, with an unpredictable and mysterious wandering womb, and without enough humoral heat to produce significant intelligence or independence. Female infants, they speculated, were the result of incomplete formation in the womb[1]. These writers came up with numerous interpretations as to why a female might be born instead of a male. Aristotle in particular thought little of women and their abilities, seeing them as beings who were limited by their imperfections. While some authors, such as those

1 This is reflective of the place/status of women in ancient Greek society. Women were usually confined to the home and sequestered from public life.

Vaughan, Theresa A., *Women, Food, and Diet in the Middle Ages: Balancing the Humours*. Taylor & Francis Group, 2020
DOI: 10.5117/9789462989382_CH03

contributing to the Hippocratic Corpus, remained more neutral in tone than Aristotle, it is clear that Greek theoretical medicine was based on the idea that women were imperfect men.

Regarding the humours, women were considered to be colder and moister than men, a condition with implications for diet and humoral balance. Humoral heat was essential to process, or 'concoct' food effectively, and women were unable to completely concoct their food. Excess noxious substances resulting from incomplete concoction were eliminated through menstruation, a natural process necessary to the maintenance of female health. Women, these authors wrote, also benefitted from the sexual act; humorally cold female bodies craved the heat of the male body. For some authors, such as Aristotle, this meant that women naturally craved sex, and were by nature wanton and impassioned in their search for a male sexual partner[2]. A cessation of the menses, or, in the medical parlance of the day "retention" of the menses, which was not due to pregnancy or menopause, was treated as a grave health hazard, for it meant that the noxious substances resulting from incomplete concoction could not be eliminated. Numerous recipes and techniques are found in the ancient and medieval medical literature that purport to counteract retention of the menses.

Physiologically, women also had the unique experience of pregnancy and childbirth. While conception and the formation of the foetus occupied the thoughts of natural philosophers, the mechanics of birth were less often the subject of scholarly inquiry. Some ancient and medieval obstetrical guides addressed different birth presentations as well as births of abnormal infants. However, the basics of helping a woman through a normal birth were typically left to midwives or female relatives, not considered important enough to comment upon (Karamanou et al. 2013).

This chapter and the next trace some of the history of medical writing about women, from Aristotle and Hippocrates to the various versions of the *Trotula* (generally positive about women) and *De secretis mulierum* (generally negative about women), as well as other sources particularly pertinent to female health, much of which focused on conception, pregnancy, and childbirth. In fact, treatises on women's health written by men are typically exclusively about gynaecology and obstetrics (Lemay 1992, 33). Within this

2 In the ancient world, chastity did not have the same overtones of virtue and sinlessness as it would after the introduction of Christianity. Virginity and then fidelity within a marriage were important primarily to secure the male line of succession. Women's craving for sex was viewed as an involuntary need to correct humoral imbalance, and maintenance of virginity or chastity within a marriage, or refusal to marry to maintain chastity, was viewed as an anomaly.

written tradition, it is possible to tease out information specifically on diet. Dietary references can be found in handbooks on women's health and physiology, as well as more general texts on health, particularly in texts like the various *Regimina sanitatis*, and versions of the *Tacuina sanitatis*. In these works, female humoral composition is considered, just as any individual's humoral composition was considered by physicians when prescribing a dietary regime. Where available, class distinctions that informed dietary recommendations are noted; however, dietary recommendations for women in the written tradition meant aristocratic women, who were thought to have a more delicate constitution.

Class, gender, diet, and humoral theory

Aristocratic women might be prescribed diets different from those of men, being 'colder' in nature (in the medical sense) than men, as their constitutions were considered the most delicate. It's possible that some form of Greek medicine made its way into folk medicine as well, but traditional ideas about food and health would have prevailed (Stannard 2013). To what extent medieval people followed these recommendations is not fully known, though archaeology and manorial records do offer some ideas (Woolgar 2010). The diet of the average person, whether peasant, aristocrat, or clergy, was also dictated by the many fast days in the Christian calendar when meat (though not fish) was forbidden. The relationship between religion and diet is explored more fully in Chapter Eight.

To briefly summarize the process described in Chapter Two, different foods were processed in a variety of ways by the body. The utility of any given foodstuff was dependent upon the nature of the food itself as well as the cooking technique used (Laurioux 2006a, 224). It was also the very nature of the body to process food into useful components depending on the complexion of the individual body itself; in humoral terms, the cold and moist complexion of women might not make effective use of the same types of food as the hot and dry complexion of men.[3] The writers in the Greco-Roman medical tradition believed that food could reconstitute into vital bodily substances (or wastes) according to its humoral nature. In its

3 These are generalizations. It was possible for individual men or women to vary in complexion, some women being hotter and drier than others, some men being hot or moist. Such variances could be interpreted as causing disease, and could be corrected through individually prescribed diet.

Christianized medical formulation, at creation everything was made out of the four elements. Food, therefore, had a humoral profile based upon its elements. Ingesting the right kind of food could address deficiencies or excesses of these elements, which translate in the body into humours. 'Blood was analogous to air, therefore it was hot and wet ... phlegm, cold and wet, is homologous to water; [yellow] bile, hot and dry, is homologous to fire; finally [black] bile, cold and dry, is homologous to the earth[4] (Jacquart 2006, 261). General guidelines existed for food consumption based upon humoral composition, but a physician was expected to understand the nature and proper balance of a patient based upon his or her complexion, and what foods might maintain or restore a proper humoral balance (Laurioux 2006b). Numerous treatises from the Middle Ages provide similar information on the proper preparation and nature of different foodstuffs for promoting health (Nicoud 2008, 8). These ideas seem to have remained fairly fixed throughout the medieval era, held not just by the learned but found in folklore and the oral tradition as well (Benedek 1978).

Aristotle

As mentioned in Chapter Two, Aristotle wrote significant treatises on natural philosophy (among his many other works), though his ideas specifically on conception and embryonic development were typically not adopted by later natural philosophers or medical authors, save for a few outliers. Rhazes, the Arabic systematist, chose to champion some of Aristotle's ideas, and Thomas Aquinas (1225-1274 CE, Roccasecca, Italy) reintroduced natural philosophical concepts from Aristotle in his own theological writing. Throughout the Middle Ages, however, Aristotle's natural philosophy was less influential than the ideas found in the Hippocratic Corpus as modified by Galen (Lemay 1992, 40).

In the Greco-Roman tradition sex and pregnancy were considered necessary for the proper functioning of the female body, which naturally craved sexual intercourse for its warming properties. Pregnancy was also a natural state, but since the normal process of eliminating noxious substances and corrupt humours through the menses was halted during this time, it was especially important that women eat foods that could be completely

4 '... le sang est homologue de l'air, car il est chaud et humide, les deux qualities caractéristique de la vie; le phlegme, froid et humide est homologue de l'eau; la bile, chaude et sèche est homologue du feu; enfin la mélancolie, froid et sèche, est homologue de la terre'. Translation my own.

concocted, minimizing the production of detrimental substances. The emphasis on the propagation of the male line in ancient Greece (as well as Rome and the later Middle Ages) meant that women were under surveillance to ensure they didn't have sex with other partners. It was essential to keep the bloodline pure (Laurent 1989, 25-27).

The Hippocratic Corpus

The Hippocratic Corpus (fifth century BCE-second century CE) contains a number of treatises on female physiology, mostly found in *The Diseases of Women* 1 and 2. Clearly not written by a single author, these collected volumes explore the health of women largely from the standpoint of gynaecological or obstetric concerns. The treatises contained in these volumes are sometimes mutually contradictory, but unlike Aristotle's works, seem to combine practical medical knowledge with theoretical models. While not as clearly formulated as they would become with Galen or later Arabic systematists, the basics of later humoral medicine are present in these volumes.

It should be noted that the Hippocratic Corpus[5] is primarily concerned with women as vehicles for gestation and childbirth. Continuation of the male line was of primary concern and women were necessary for the continuation of that line. It is likely that this cultural emphasis influenced the obstetrical orientation of the HC. In addition, the reproductive system was the primary way in which the female body differed anatomically from the male body. The Hippocratic writings are not as openly hostile to women as some of the works of Aristotle; nevertheless, the Greek cultural attitude towards women is still very much present.

Works specific to women from the HC surviving into the Middle Ages and beyond were the *Eight-Month Child, Generating Seed/Nature of the Child, Diseases of Women* (in two books), *Barren Women, Nature of Women, Superfetation, Young Girls*, and *Excision of the Embryo*. Taken together, these treatises cover a wide range of topics pertinent to obstetrics and gynaecology, including both concerns of natural philosophy (embryonic development) and medicine (menstruation, infertility, contraception, and mechanics of birth, among other topics).

The recipes in the HC are sometimes for the making of medicine, but are often dietary recommendations to aid in healing. For example, in a section of *Diseases of Women 1*, the author outlines a procedure for helping women

5 Referred to hereafter as HC

conceive when conception has proven difficult. Among the treatments – which involve the woman lying still for up to thirty days to prevent the male seed from leaving the womb – are recommendations for diet. During the first week after intercourse, while she lies still, the infertile woman should drink unsalted barley groats in water but take no solid food. While the author does not explain the theoretical basis for this recommendation, barley was considered a very easily digested food, thus leaving no residue which would result in excess menstrual blood.[6] The patient is also instructed not to bathe, thus preventing the semen from being washed out of the womb. The exact role of semen in conception was a matter for debate, but physicians and natural philosophers recognized that it had a key role in conception. After seven days the patient may eat wheat bread or barley cakes, poultry or fish (whichever one settles the stomach), should not eat bitter vegetables, should drink dark red wine, and should have her meat baked rather than boiled, perhaps so as not to add extra moisture (Hanson 1975, 579). Red wine also has heating and drying properties. The dietary recommendations make sense within the scope of humoral theory, as well as the cultural constraints of what was readily available and part of the local diet.

Soranus of Ephesus

It is likely that Soranus of Ephasus received his medical training in Alexandria, and later practiced in Rome. He was a prolific author who addressed gynaecology and obstetrics in his work *Gynaecology* (*On Midwifery and the Diseases of Women*). Soranus was the best-known obstetrician in antiquity, though his work was not taken up in the Arabic world, unlike the works of Galen and to a lesser extent Aristotle. As a result, Soranus' work did not pass into European Latin translation by the twelfth century, when medicine underwent rapid professionalization (Lemay 1992, 38). He wrote specifically about midwives, and *Gynaecology* is one of the texts providing some understanding of midwifery in the ancient world. Soranus set out guidelines for what makes a qualified midwife: she 'must be able to read and write; she must have a thorough knowledge of the theory and practice of obstetrics and she must be experienced in all areas of medicine as to give dietetic as well as surgical and pharmacological prescriptions' (Karamanou et al. 2013, 227). A midwife should also keep her nails trimmed so as to

6 Barley water continues to be considered healthful for invalids and upset stomachs in the folk medicine of some areas of Europe to this day.

avoid wounding female organs, be discreet and keep secrets, and should not believe in spirits or other things of a superstitious[7] nature. Finally, she should not be greedy nor too eager to sell abortifacients, for which there seems to have been a consistent demand.

Soranus recommended that properly trained midwives should attend uncomplicated births, with a (male) physician only being called in for complicated cases. He also wrote about the choice of a proper wet nurse and suggested a diet that a wet nurse should follow to produce healthy milk for an infant. Soranus also had specific dietary recommendations for pregnant women, counselling the consumption of 'neutral foods,' such as non-greasy meats or fish and non-pungent vegetables. Conversely, the patient should avoid pungent vegetables, preserved meats and fish, and very moist foods (Matalas, Zampelas, and Stavrinos 2001, 15). Among the conditions of pregnancy he addressed with dietary recommendations were pica (geophagia), nausea, and vomiting.

The reasoning behind Soranus' dietary recommendations are not made clear, but, like the HC, also reflects a combination of humoral properties of foodstuffs as well as culturally appropriate and readily available items. While both Soranus' *Gynaecology* and the HC make recommendations typical of a Mediterranean diet, they do reflect the culinary differences between Greece and Rome. Soranus was one of the 'Methodist' medical writers of his day. For medical Methodists[8], diseases either required surgery or dietetic and pharmacological treatment. Dietetic diseases involved excessively dry and constricted states (*status strictus*), excessively fluid and atonic states (*status laxus*), or a combination (*status mixtus*). Dietary advice was geared towards mitigating the deleterious consequences of these states (Drabkin 1951, 505).

Galen of Pergamum

Galen of Pergamum, previously discussed, was perhaps the single greatest influence on medieval European medicine. Unlike Soranus, however, Galen wrote no single work on gynaecology that survives; in fact, his works rarely address gynaecology at all. Galen was an amazingly prolific author. A few

7 'Superstitious' is a value-laden term typically not used in the study of folk or traditional belief, but it is a more exact translation of the word used by Soranus.

8 The Methodic school of medical thought focused on knowledge of the disease only as the key to finding the appropriate cure. Methodist physicians thought the cause of the disease was irrelevant.

of his treatises are specific to gynaecological concerns, such as *De uteri dissectione* (*On the Dissection of the Uterus*), and *De foetuum formatione* (*On the Formation of the Foetus*), but these works are less about the treatment of women and more about anatomy (in the former) and natural philosophy and embryology (in the latter). There are references to women throughout the surviving corpus, and Galen certainly elaborated upon on the humoral theory initially described in the HC.

Despite the dearth of gynaecological treatises, Galen's development of medical treatments and the role of diet in maintenance of health and treatment of disease is instrumental to understanding some of the later work specific to women. Galen made dietary recommendations for many illnesses. His recommendations for dietary treatment based on humoral theory are available in their most detailed form in *De alimentorum facultatibus* (*On the Powers of Foods*) and in other works on hygiene, as well as in *De facultatibus naturalibus* (*On the Natural Faculties*). There are, of course, many other treatises by Galen which mention diet and humoral theory, or make recommendations that may be appropriate to women.

We know that Galen's works were part of the medical curriculum at the School of Alexandria, and that they also became part of the rise of university-trained physicians translated through the Arabic systematists. In fact, it was these systematists, attempting to synthesize and organize medical theory from Hippocrates, Galen, Aristotle, and other Greco-Roman sources, who 'reframed non-Galenic material about women's disorders within a Galenic explanation of female humoral physiology' (Wallis 2010, 185). So, while later European medical writers owed a significant debt to Galen for the medieval foundations of theoretical medicine and the importance of diet, he actually gave very few specific recommendations for the treatment of women.

The Islamic texts of the Arabic systematists

Ibn al-Jazzār, Latinized as Algizar, (895-979 CE, Kairouan) was a medieval scholar born in Tunisia, the nephew of the more famous Abu Bakr. Algizar lived an austere life, and apparently did not look for a position in one of the princely courts. He saw patients and examined their urine for free,[9]

9 Examination of the urine was an extremely common method of diagnosis, or aid in diagnosis of many diseases. It was so common that quack physicians examining urine show up in fabliaux and other popular entertainments. Illuminated manuscripts and some medical texts also depict

also dispensing medicine for free. He wrote many treatises on a variety of subjects, but focused especially on medicine. Algizar's works, like that of a number of Arabic writers, were known in medieval Western Europe. He produced a medical handbook drawing on the works of a number of Greco-Roman authors, including Aristotle, Hippocrates, and Galen, entitled *Zad al Mussafir*, known in Europe as the *Viaticum*. The *Viaticum* was translated into Greek early on, translated into Hebrew multiple times, and finally translated into Latin. It was widely used in medical schools and universities. One section was on women's diseases, and it became a primary source for one of the *Trotula* treatises. Algizar drew some of the text of the *Viaticum* from Galen and the seventh-century Paul of Aegina (c. 625-c. 690 CE). Evidence for Galen's ideas on humoral pathology are found in his work (Bos 1993).

Like a number of authors before him, Algizar wrote about menstruation's central role in maintaining female health. Irregular or absent menstruation caused diseases in women. Algizar followed the Greek interpretation that the menses are the result of women's cold nature, which meant they could only incompletely digest or concoct their food, with the resulting waste material expelled during the menses. Algizar also, like the Greeks, subscribed to the natural inferiority of women. As symptoms of amenorrhoea, in addition to the retention of the menses, the *Viaticum* cites lack of appetite, nausea, and craving for substances that are unnatural to eat – such as charcoal and earth[10]. The remedies he prescribed incorporated pharmaceuticals, decoctions, fumigations, and suppositories, typical treatments in the works of Galen. Algizar likewise addressed hypermenorrhoea, or excessive blood loss during menstruation, as well as 'suffocation' of the uterus – meaning displacement of the uterus[11] – the idea that problems could arise when the womb wandered from its original position, affecting the other organs (Bos 1993). Algizar also outlined a dietary regimen for pregnant women very similar to that of Galen.

A number of the Arabic systematists wrote about proper nutrition for pregnant women, and their recommendations are likely the source of the later versions of the *Regimen sanitatis*. One of the best known of the Arabic systematists was Rhazes. Rhazes' *Liber de medicine ad Almansorem* (c. CE

the examination of urine by doctors, and provide guidelines to medical students about what to look for to make a diagnosis.

10 This condition is still recognized today, known as *pica* or geophagia.

11 The concept of the 'wandering womb' came from the Greeks, who believed the womb could literally become unmoored from its location, wandering to other parts of the body. It is from this concept that we get the term 'hysteria' for a nervous condition considered especially common in women.

903) included a section on dietary regimes for women and small children: *De regimene infantis et pregnantis*. This section was just one of several that included recommendations for care of women in childbirth, childcare, and choice of a suitable wet nurse. For pregnant women, Rhazes advised against consuming anything that might provoke an abortion or menstruation, such as pungent and bitter foods, as well as any activities which might do likewise. A pregnant woman should avoid being bled, exercising too vigorously, taking long baths, staying too long in the sun, or having sexual intercourse. Rhazes' food recommendations are common to nearly all texts – light and easily digestible foods, especially poultry (Weiss-Amer 1992, 307). He was well-versed in Greco-Roman medicine, and even wrote a treatise taking issue with some of Galen's ideas, entitled 'Doubts About Galen'.

Another prominent Islamic writer, Avicenna, was the author of *Canon medicinae*. This Arabic text became a leading textbook in European medical schools after its translation into Latin in the mid-1100s. Preventative medicine is an important part of this work, which also included much on the identification and treatment of disease. Avicenna's work included a consideration of sexuality and reproductive organs, as well as dietary regimes for conception and birth, pregnancy, wet-nurses, and a discussion of the appetite of pregnant women. His dietary recommendations for pregnancy are very similar to those in Rhazes' *Liber de medicine ad Almansorem* (Weiss-Amer 1992, 308).

Most European-authored regimes for pregnancy followed the advice of Rhazes and Avicenna, with occasional additions from the HC or Galen. Thus, the Islamic writers, or Arabic Systematists, organized and systematized the Greco-Roman medical treatises that made it into the Islamic work. The Systematists' work would begin to be available in Europe around the eleventh century, just as European medical schools were being established.

The *Trotula*

In the late eleventh and into the twelfth centuries, Salerno – a port city in what is now Italy – was an early outpost of the Western European professionalization of medicine, with a reputation for having an excellent medical school. Reputedly, one female physician both practiced and taught medicine in the school of Salerno, a Dame Trota (or Trot, or Trocta), and a collection of writings came to be attributed to her. The general trend of scholarly opinion is that a woman of Salerno associated with the name Trota was active in medicine in the twelfth century (Stuard 1975). While Trota's existence and authorship are somewhat in doubt,[12] there is evidence that such a person practiced medicine, and that she either wrote down, or her students wrote down, some of her teachings (Green 2002). The *Trotula* is focused almost exclusively on female health and reproductive medicine.

The *Trotula* contains three distinct parts. While it is highly unlikely that all three treatises (*Liber de sinthomatibus mulierum* or *Book on the Conditions of Women, De curis mulierum* or *On Treatments for Women*, and *De ornatu mulierum* or *On Women's Cosmetics*) were written by Trota, Green (2002) argues convincingly that *On Treatments for Women* was likely based upon Trota's ideas, either through her own writing or a record of her teaching (2002, 49-50).

Drawing on Galen and the Arabic systematists, whose work would have been known in this Italian port city, the *Trotula* is not the earliest work out of the Salernitan school of medicine, but it is unique in its exclusive focus on women, as well as its combination of both practical treatments and theoretical medicine. The work was considered so important that its texts or fragments of its texts can be found through the sixteenth century, as far away as England (Rowland 1981). There are many dietary recommendations for women's health and treatment of disease within the three treatises of the *Trotula,* and these are treated in much greater detail in Chapter Five.

Hildegard of Bingen

Hildegard of Bingen, mentioned previously, was a German abbess who wrote music, was a visionary, and who also wrote widely on theology, science, and medicine. She is unusual for being one of the few woman authors known from the twelfth century whose authorship of most of the works attributed to her is not seriously in dispute. While very influential in her own region, her work was less widely read and had much less influence on the history of medicine in Europe than the *Trotula*. While Hildegard clearly demonstrated considerable knowledge of the written Latin tradition, her understanding of medicine and health were rather idiosyncratic – filtered through the lens of her own theology – from which her medical works are inseparable. Additionally, Hildegard may only have had access to a limited number of Latin medical texts. She was primarily remembered as a visionary and

12 Scholarly opinion runs the gamut from an insistence that she was a real individual who wrote all three treatises of the *Trotula*, to insistence that there is no evidence of her existence and the name is simply that of a fictional female doctor that became attached to the texts.

composer. While Hildegard did not write a treatise solely on women's health, two of her works incorporate medicine and natural philosophy, and include some specific recommendations for women. Hildegard viewed herself as a visionary inspired by God, which may have given her more license to stray from practical matters and speculate on the relationship of God to humankind (Green 2008, 68). Influential figures of her time, most notably Bernard of Clairvaux, attested to her status as a visionary to the Vatican.

The two books most pertinent to food and medicine are *Physica* (1998) and *Causae et curae* (1999, 2006). These works are not solely about medicine *per se*, but include an assessment of the humoral nature and properties of many plants, animals, and potentially edible substances (*Physica*), as well as general medical advice (*Causae et Curae*) based on her interpretation of humoral composition and how it may be corrected. Hildegard's understanding of the humoral system varied somewhat from what was taught in medical schools, and that understanding is reflected in her writing. For example, she describes the four qualities as 'dry, wet, tepid, and foamy' (Marron 2014), as opposed to hot, cold, moist, and dry. The theological argument presented in these works was intended to demonstrate that the human body is a microcosm of God's creation, and that understanding the body helps us to better understand God. There is no evidence that Hildegard was a trained physician, though it has been argued that she would have known about both folk medicine and some Greco-Roman medicine, and that she may have served as a medicus for the abbey and surrounding area (Sweet 2006).

Hildegard is discussed in greater depth in Chapter Five, focusing on her diet advice found primarily in *Causae et curae.* While Hildegard's suggested treatment of diseases was comprised mostly of plant-based medicine, she did offer advice on diet as well as occasional regimens specific to women's concerns. Hildegard had a very definite view of procreation within the realm of creation, viewing it as a blessing by God (though perhaps not as perfect a state as virginity), but did not incorporate much Christian moralizing into the writing of the text itself. In contrast, on the rather extreme end of judgement of women as sexual beings, we have our next text, *De secretis mulierum.*

De secretis mulierum

De secretis mulierum (c. 1300 CE) was attributed to Albertus Magnus (1193-1280 CE, Lauingen, Germany), but clearly was not written by him. It is currently attributed to "pseudo-Albertus," as we do not know the original author. *De secretis mulierum* is essentially a book on natural philosophy, focusing on procreation, ostensibly written for celibate monks. In one of the surviving one hundred or so manuscripts, based primarily on the Lyons 1508 edition and translated by Lemay (1992), the original text is supplemented by the opinions of two commentators addressing the statements of the text itself, occasionally contradicting, but more often simply adding further confirmative information and commentary. Pseudo-Albertus is heir to the tradition of Aristotle, more so than that of Galen, though elements of Galen are found in the work. While Galen was not exactly a proto-feminist, his work was less actively hostile to women than that of Aristotle. Pseudo-Albertus, and his commentators, are quite clearly anti-feminist. Females are portrayed as having an impure nature (Lemay 1992, 47). For pseudo-Albertus, as for Aristotle and his heirs, women are deformed men, and their menstrual blood is filthy and poisonous, worse than the most corrosive poison. Menstrual flow, according to the commentators, could back up into the eyes, and those eyes could poison others with just a glance, because the menstrual poison could poison the air, and the poisonous air could infect others.

Menstrual taboos are common in world cultures. Menstruation is sometimes seen as polluting, and therefore dangerous to men, crops, or to the group as a whole. Anthropologists have noted the cultural practices surrounding menstruation for many cultures, and how menstrual practices are part of daily activities. More often than not, cultural perceptions of menstruation are negative. In some cases, women are not permitted to cook for their husbands or families for fear of poisoning the food or rendering it unwholesome. In notable examples, women have to remove themselves from the family home, spending time in a designated structure for menstruating women until their periods end. It is also common to be forbidden from visiting sacred places, or to wear some visible sign of the fact that she is menstruating. There have been many interpretations for why this should be so culturally universal, but none are accepted as telling the whole story (Small 1999). The ancient Greeks, the source of medical concern here with menstrual blood, were certainly not alone. However, Greek attitudes towards menstruation and the female body are here read through the anti-feminist tradition in ecclesiastical writing.

According to pseudo-Albertus, 'Woman is less suited to morals than man, for the humidity of her complexion is easily mobile, thus she is inconstant and always seeking something new. Thus, if she were having sex with one man, if it were possible, she would want to be with another at the same time. Consequently, there is no faith in woman, and a sign of this is that wise men tell their wives as little as possible about their words and deeds.

Woman is thus a failed man, with a defective nature' (Lemay 1992, 48). This could have been taken straight from Aristotle, whose views tended to be more popular among ecclesiastical authors than strictly medical authors. The author then goes on to connect women with the devil, attributing to them evil plots, poison, and deviousness to obtain what they want.

De secretis mulierum does offer the standard advice and explanations linking menstruation and diet. With the text and the commentaries taken together in the Lyons 1508 edition, the following dietary advice is offered: women who consume delicate and highly spiced foods can expect subtler menstrual flow, while poor women who eat course or inferior quality foods can expect the opposite. Pregnant women are highly desirous of sex because they take in superfluous matter (food) without the usual remedy of it being expelled through the menses, and the heat from this excess matter inflames the vulva, making women crave the heat of sexual intercourse. Sexual intercourse should be undertaken on an empty stomach, because a body digesting food will have heat transferred from the digesting organs to the reproductive organs – thus having sex on a full stomach will impair digestion. Flax seed cooked in camel's milk acts as an aphrodisiac when eaten, while lettuce seed and lentils boiled together, when consumed, lessens the libido (Lemay 1992, 69-77). In short, *De Secretis Mulierum* is not really a book on women's health, nor a health regimen for women, but simply a work of anti-feminist natural philosophy.

Regimina sanitatis and *Tacuina sanitatis*

A number of *Regimina sanitatis* (rules of health) were written with recommendations intended for women. Many were derived largely from the work of Arabic writers and systematists, such as Johannitius, Haly Abbas, Rhazes, and Avicenna. Ultimately, most health recommendations in the *Regimen sanitatis* can be traced back to the humoral theory of the HC and Galen, as with much of medieval medical thought. These guides included not only recommendations for diet, but for all of the six 'non-naturals'.[13] The intent of these regimens was to give advice about remaining healthy or treating certain kinds of illness. According to Weiss-Amer (1992, 302), three states were addressed in these books: health, illness, and a neutral state. The neutral state included those who weren't ill, but whose health was precarious or

13 The six non-naturals are: air, food and drink, exercise and rest, sleep and waking, repletion and excretion, and the passions and emotions.

delicate. Individuals in this neutral state were pregnant women, children, the convalescing, and the elderly. In fact, dietary advice for everyone in this neutral group remained fairly similar.

The monk Heinrich Laufenberg, (CE 1391-1460, Freiburg) completed a *Regimen* in 1429, the first written in the German vernacular. It included among its seven parts a general *Regimen sanitatis* for healthy adults, primarily men, but also one for pregnant women and young children. Laufenberg's work was somewhat unusual in that it did not cover certain aspects of women's health, such as conception and childbirth, ostensibly because these were subjects the Church considered inappropriate topics for monks. In his prologue, Laufenberg made clear his approach: 'pregnancy is a state blessed by God, women are delicate creatures who need to be given proper – male – advice, and the health of both mother and child are important' (Weiss-Amer 1992, 304). He advised caution in more than just dietary choices. A pregnant woman should not experience strong emotions, she should clear her mind of worries, avoid physical trauma, and be given good food and drink, as she desired.

As had become the norm, the general dietary advice given for pregnant women was similar to that given to all people in fragile health. According to Laufenberg, pregnant women should eat delicate and easily concocted foods such as veal, lamb, chicken, partridge, other small fowl, venison, and soft-boiled eggs. As delivery approached, one of the dishes Laufenberg recommended was hot milk or mush. After giving birth, a woman's diet should include poultry and light white wine. Foods to be avoided included those more difficult to completely concoct, such as beef, pork, smoked meats, beans, lentils, barley, raw fruit and certain kinds of fish. (Weiss-Amer 1992, 306) Some of the food cautioned against was thought of as coarse or tough, some overly warming (beef or pork) and some overly cold (fresh fruits, certain kinds of fish). There was a humoral basis for these recommendations; complete concoction would prevent excess bleeding in the postpartum period, as there would be less humoral waste to expel. It is important to note, however, that the diet also included food considered delicate and appropriate for upper-class people, thought to be suited for refined and light foods. Note also the changes in specific food recommendations from those of ancient Greece, such as the recommendation here against barley and fish, demonstrating culture-based food preferences and food availability. This is one instance among many where it is clear that local and traditional regional dietary patterns and beliefs have affected literate culture – an example of folk beliefs influencing theoretical medicine.

Another European regimen written in the vernacular was the *Régime du corps*, by Aldobrandin of Siena[14] (d. c. 1296 CE). This thirteenth-century Italian physician was resident in France from 1277 until his death in 1296. The French text included a regime for pregnant women based largely on the work of Avicenna (Weiss-Amer 1992, 309). Aldobrandin also took his cue from important Arabic authors and added his own suggestions for pregnant women. For example, Aldobrandin advised against consuming salty food and foods that provoked frequent urination. A pregnant woman should eat moderate and well-balanced meals including good meats and good wine diluted with water. Pears, ginger, cardamom and muscat nut could be consumed to comfort the stomach when the pregnant woman was feeling nauseous (Laurent 1989, 126).

Valascus de Tarenta (d. 1417 CE), active in the late fourteenth and early fifteenth centuries, was another physician resident in France at the medical school of Montpellier. Valascus authored a *Regimine pregnantium* as well. He advised pregnant women to avoid highly spiced dishes, capers, unripe olives, beans, sesame, wild mint, and horseradish. Instead, pregnant women should eat good food, drink old red wine, eat fresh eggs, and ripe fruit such as pear or quince. Elements of Valascus' regimen that involved other 'non-naturals' were also included: a pregnant woman should not bathe too much, get too much sun, work too hard, exercise too much, or be exposed to too much cold, damp air. She should think pleasant thoughts and smell nice things (Laurent 1989, 126-127). Here again, these recommendations probably stem, at least in part, from folk beliefs.

The *Tacuinum sanitatis* is a variation on the *Regimen sanitatis* that exists in a number of different versions, with the four most complete manuscripts from late fourteenth century Lombardy, though much earlier versions exist. It is based on the *Taqwim as-sinhah* (Maintenance of Health), an eleventh-century manuscript by the Christian physician Ibn Butlan of Baghdad (1001-1038 CE). The *Tacuinum* seems to be a cross between an herbal[15] and a *Regimen sanitatis*. It lists dietary guidelines and environmental factors that can affect health. It is not arranged alphabetically, as an herbal would be; rather, its arrangement reflects the components of a normal diet. The extant copies are heavily illustrated, and unlike herbals, show plants growing in their natural habitats with people eating, preparing, and cultivating them. The *Tacuinum sanitatis* is clearly intended for a lay audience rather than

14 In French, Aldebrandin de Sienne.

15 A guide to plants and herbs, listed alphabetically by species name, and often illustrated/illuminated.

for trained physicians. Its illustrations are suggestive of 'Labours of the Months' (Henisch 1995), but developed just for these manuscripts. A variety of social classes are shown, each eating or doing things typical for that class. Women are frequently depicted in these illustrations. Essentially, the books focus on the six non-naturals. Recommendations for women's health and diet are not as explicit as in the *Regimina sanitatis* mentioned above, but the depiction of women preparing and consuming certain foods, as well as participating in various activities, can give us some specific ideas about regimens for women's health (Witthoft 1978).

Michele Savonarola

A later health manuscript, *De regimine pregnantium,* was written by Michele Savonarola (1385-1468, Padua) in the fifteenth century. Savonarola, as most authors before him, classified women as cold and moist. As noted above, in Greek medicine women were viewed medically as imperfect men. Savonarola took a slightly more neutral stance, but while he didn't pathologize pregnancy, he did view the state of pregnancy as one requiring special dietary treatment similar to that of a convalescent patient, which was common in the written tradition (Marafioti 2010, 21). Savonarola's unique contribution was to take complicated and technical Latin texts and simplify them into the local vernacular (in this case, of Ferrara) so that medical texts were accessible to literate women of the city. He posited that women could help determine the sex of their children (in favour of an all-important boy child) by consuming warm and dry foods (according to humoral theory). 'Savonarola sustains that the warmth and dryness of certain foods will cancel out a woman's inferior qualities and shape the foetus into a robust and healthy male child' (Marafioti 2010, 26).

Desire for male offspring and the continuation of family lines was common in all cultures, but at particular instances reached points of more emphasis and anxiety. This was especially important for the nobility and monied classes, as being able to pass down inherited titles and/or wealth would become an imperative of maintaining social class and prominence. This would be true of the Early Modern period as well, and later into the twentieth century. In fact, concerns over fertility for the upper classes were manifest in multiple regions of Europe: France (Bavaye-Kouidrat 2016), Italy (Androniki 2011), and England (Toulalan 2014), to name a few.

Savonarola recommended that women eat three times a day, rather than the twice a day customary for middle- and upper-class people. He listed meats of animals (four-leggeds), poultry (two-leggeds) and fish, weighing both their beneficial and harmful aspects. 'He recommends moderation above all else, stressing that foods that are too cold or moist should be avoided. Since women were thought to be excessively cold and moist by nature, it was especially important for expectant mothers to counterbalance the qualities of their nutritional intake with those of their own temperament" (Marafioti 2010, 30).

For example, fish, considered a cold and moist food, should be eaten only in small quantities by a pregnant woman, and only those who tended to a choleric (hot) or sanguine (dry) temperament, and then only if properly prepared. For those women Savonarola recommended that fish be roasted or cooked in wine, with cinnamon or salt in order to reduce its cold and moist properties. Wine and fire were considered warming, and cinnamon or salt had drying properties. He cautioned against eating fried fish, as he (as well as Galen) considered fried foods appropriate for healthy individuals, but not for pregnant women, who were placed into the same category as invalids and convalescents (Marafioti 2010, 30). We begin to get an idea of what particular foods were recommended when we examine recipe collections from this time, such as in the work of Maestro Martino or other attributed authors of the late medieval period (Notaker 2017).

Other writers

Arnaldus de Villa Nova (1235-1311), a thirteenth century physician from Valencia or Aragon who taught at the medical school in Montpellier, was a prolific author who wrote on female health and sexuality. He noted that sterility 'comes about when the woman is too unpleasant, malicious and overheated in thought'[16] (Laurent 1989, 47). Arnaldus also believed that an improper dietary regime could hinder conception, when the woman 'eats meats which are too sharp or sour or when she is in the habit of eating poor quality meat'[17] (Laurent 1989, 51). To ease birth, Arnaldus prescribed bay leaf in wine (Laurent 1989, 188); for pain after childbirth, he suggested raw egg cooked in white wine.

While there is less evidence available for Hebrew treatments of obstetrics compared to the Arab world or medieval Europe, some do exist

16 'vent quand la femme set trop mauvaise, malicieuse et cogitative en pensée'. Translation my own.

17 'mange viandes trop aigres ou qu'elle a costume de manger viande de mauvaise qualité'. Translation my own.

(Caballero-Navas 2008). We know that there was an exchange of knowledge between Muslim, Christian, and Jewish cultures; however, we know less than we might because surviving Hebrew obstetric texts remain relatively unstudied and mostly untranslated. Early medieval Jewish medical literature was often written in Arabic, or sometimes Judeo-Arabic (Arabic written with Hebrew letters). One Jewish medical author is Seset ben Yitzhaq ben Yosef Benveniste (1131-1209), who was born in Narbonne and practiced in Barcelona. Two of his works still survive, *Medicament for pregnancy*, and *Medicaments and confections for women's diseases* (Barkai 1988, 99). There are also a number of surviving texts by unknown authors. One such work is the *Book of Dina* (date unknown). Several of these treatises, though traceable to other sources of influence, tend to contain more material from the Hebrew scriptures than the Christian *New Testament* or Muslim texts. One work, an illuminated manuscript fragment entitled *Miqosi ha-Leda* (*On Difficulties of Birth*) exists in a fourteenth century manuscript. While not containing an abundance of dietary advice, it is notable in that it goes over many different kinds of fetal malpresentation[18], with illustrations. Some of this work may derive from the *Gynaecology* of Soranus (Barkai 1988).

Non-medical texts and folk beliefs

Les Quinze Joies de Mariage (*The Fifteen Joys of Marriage*) is a late fourteenth- or fifteenth-century anonymous satirical text in the anti-feminist tradition that portrays the trials and tribulations of marriage, and mocks men who are not in control of their own households. While not addressing a specific regime during pregnancy, it does portray women as becoming mentally unbalanced during pregnancy. The text advises that women be given whatever they want to eat during pregnancy, and gently talked out of things not good for them (Laurent 1989, 128).

Le Miroir de Mariage (*The Mirror of Marriage*) is another satirical text, this time by a known author, Eustache Deschamps (1346-1406, Champagne). Written around the year 1400, it is a satirical poem on the subject of women. Deschamps became well known during his lifetime, and *Le Miroir de Mariage* was one of the inspirations for Chaucer's work. The text reflects the common folk belief that the unsatisfied cravings and wild imaginations of pregnant women could impact a developing foetus. For example, if a pregnant woman desired cherries, strawberries, or wine, and her cravings

18 A malpresentation is when a baby is positioned for birth in an abnormal manner.

remained unfulfilled, the child might be born with a red or port-wine birthmark. The poem also reflects the idea that what a woman consumed during pregnancy could affect her foetus. For example, she shouldn't eat soft cheese, because if she had a boy, he would have a short life. If she had a girl, she would be ugly. If a small child was wanted, she should eat toasted white bread soaked in wine (Laurent 1989, 28-129).

We find some of the same ideas reflected in another composition, mentioned earlier. The *Distaff Gospels*, or *Les Evangiles des Quenouilles*, exists in several versions, the most extensive of which uses the device of a frame narrative to list the 'gospels' of a group of older women as they meet for successive nights in the presence of a clerk, who offers to write down their wisdom for posterity. These women are, of course, comic caricatures of old women, portrayed in familiar tropes as old, ugly, horny, gossips, some of whom dabble in magic and practice dubious medicine. Madeleine Jeay argues that the actual gospels of these women are very likely to be an accurate recording of folk beliefs from fifteenth century Picardie (1982).

The *Distaff Gospels* contains two types of medical advice: the first is concerned with pregnancy, and the second offers more general recommendations for health. A pregnant woman, the reader is told, should avoid eating hare's head, otherwise her child may be born with a harelip. She should not be given fish heads, which may cause a child with a large, turned-up mouth. Soft cheese should be avoided because 'if she carries a boy, he will have a short small member, and if it is a girl, her crack will be wide, deep and lean' (Garay and Jeay 2007, 429). A pregnant woman must be able to indulge her cravings, for if she does not get what she wants, the baby will be born with a mark on its body (probably in the shape of the food). Marks can also appear on a child's body if cherries, strawberries, or red wine are thrown in the face of the woman (Garay and Jeay 2007, 430). The *Distaff Gospels* are discussed further in Chapter Four.

Please note that all of these recommendations are seen in other documents, such as the *Miroir de Mariage* or Laufenburg's *Regimen,* and have the hallmarks of folk medicine. It is common, in accordance with the principles of sympathetic magic, to believe that like influences like. This concept was first explicated in terms of folklore by James George Frazer in the late 1800s, but has been an accepted principle of folk medicine for centuries before that (Frazer 1999 [1895]). It can be used to prescribe traditional medicines, and there is evidence for this principle in herbals and in the written medical tradition. It also explains the very common belief that what one eats during pregnancy (as well as what one experiences) can directly affect the baby as birthmarks or birth defects, however minor.

If we consider social class, aristocratic women were expected to be given a meal which included meat to strengthen them after birth. The meal often included a glass of wine, poultry, and bouillon in a bowl. In one case, in a painting of the Virgin after the birth of Jesus, Mary is given pâté en croute[19]! For the well to do in Tuscany, there were often special trays, called *Desco da porta,* intended just for this occasion (Musacchio 1999). Delicacies were also sent to a new mother, both for her own consumption but also to entertain visitors with fine dishes. So much was spent on this feasting after birth in the upper classes that the authorities became concerned about the extravagance. In *Le Chevalier de La Tour Landry,* written c. 1372 by Geoffroy IV de la Tour Landry (1330-1402) to his daughters to teach them proper behaviour, Geoffroy instructs his daughters about a queen who spent so lavishly on celebratory birth parties that God was displeased and her infant died. In *Le Quinze Joies de Mariage,* mentioned above, a postpartum wife wants her husband to cook for her, something of an inversion of social roles. It was a time, perhaps, when women were permitted to demand of husbands work they normally did themselves (Laurent 1989, 207-214). For example, a young wife who had newly given birth demanded a 'bon coulis de chappon au sucre' or a fine dish of chicken broth or ground chicken with sugar, a dish that came to be known as 'blancmange', a common food for invalids (Vigarello 1993, 42).

As noted previously, it is important to remember that the medical recommendations and culinary practices listed here were applicable primarily to aristocratic women. They might have applied generally to all women, with some adjustments based upon the more delicate and refined constitutions of the aristocracy and haute bourgeoisie, but the key point here is that it was generally wealthier women with the means to summon doctors and obtain their dietary advice, or afford books advising on diet and health after printing became widespread in the sixteenth century. Opening a window into the lives of average people is more challenging. There were some allowances made, perhaps, for better food before or after birth, but the medieval diet for peasants was itself rather monotonous (Montanari 2012; Ferrières 2007). Pregnant women were not necessarily treated as especially delicate. We see these dietary recommendations for women from a limited view. We also don't know, even for those who could afford the advice of a trained doctor, how likely it was for these guidelines to be followed. We know that humoral theory certainly held sway from the ancient Greeks through the Islamic world, medieval Europe, and beyond, but did people regularly practice what they were taught? Would this information in some

19 Pâté cooked in a pastry crust.

form have been circulated as part of folk medicine? This seems likely. With all we know about medicine today, compliance with medically-ordered diets is still spotty at best.

We do have some evidence of the practices of the poor. We know that theriac was a popular cure-all during the Middle Ages for those who could afford it. It was originally developed in ancient Greece as an antidote to snake bites, eventually developing into a nostrum to cure anything from asthma to poisoning (particularly for those who may be worried about being deliberately poisoned by others). Similar to hypocras, or spiced wine, it might include snake venom, believed to make the person who consumed it strong and immune to poisoning[20]. Some recipes list more than one hundred ingredients and required the concoction to be aged for twelve years or more to reach peak efficacy. The humble had to make do with other items to prevent their flesh from being corrupted by bad air or tainted water. Sailors were given onions to eat on voyages, though garlic was considered to be the 'theriac of the peasant'. Both rich and poor alike yearned for health and prevention of sickness, which could be accessed through what they consumed, be it food or medicine (Vigarello 1993, 37-39).

How can we access the dietary practices of medieval people of all social classes? In part, that question is addressed in Chapter Four, but various approaches may prove helpful – foodways, historical anthropology, archaeology, and art history may give us more information than that available in manuscripts, or at least help us interpret some of the written history. There is evidence in a few texts that can be linked back to folk medicine and the use of traditional remedies for certain conditions. For the most part, however, this is indirect evidence. Within the written tradition, we have the medical texts and medical traditions arising from the ancient Greeks and continuing on through the Middle Ages and beyond. Within that tradition, diet and treatments for women are developed according to humoral theory, with dietary recommendations comprising part of medical treatment.

In Chapter Four, we build upon the literature discussed here for a more complete distinction between theoretical and practical medicine in the treatment and dietary recommendations for women. A distinction must be made between the theoretical medicine of academically trained doctors (beginning with the Salerno school) and the practical medicine of midwives and traditional healers. By the later Middle Ages, midwives were

20 Recipes for making theriac varied, but could include a variety of substances, including herbs, honey, powdered mummy, viper flesh, spices, and opium. In England, treacle served as the theriac of the common people.

in competition with academically trained doctors for both the aristocracy and the bourgeoise, and, by the Early Modern period, would face competition from physicians even for uncomplicated births. The practical folk medicine of lay-midwives and traditional healers is, of course, more difficult to document as it was not primarily a written tradition. However, medical folklore and the literature on the anthropology of medicine offer insights into some of the differences between theoretical and practical medicine.

4 Theoretical Medicine vs. Practical Medicine

Abstract

This chapter examines the differences between theoretical medicine, empirical medicine (or medicine as practiced), and folk medicine. A particular focus on midwives and traditional healers will be enhanced by examining folklore, herbals, and other diverse examples where we can find evidence of traditional medicine. Examples of contemporary debates between traditional healing and mainstream medicine may help us sort out the different medical traditions of the Middle Ages.

Keywords: theoretical medicine, empirical medicine, practical medicine, folk medicine, medical folklore, anthropology of medicine

The previous two chapters are largely based on the Greco-Roman tradition of theoretical medicine, featuring texts outlining the practice of theoretical medicine with a focus on individual dietetics. While one can look at the recommendations in these texts and see the line of reasoning stretching from Hippocrates to the *Regimina sanitatis*, it is a much more difficult proposition to separate theoretical medicine – both *physica* and *medicina*[1] – from practical medicine. By practical medicine, I mean both medicine as actually practiced by professional doctors, and practiced by midwives, wise women, and traditional health specialists, both male and female. This practical medicine could be highly influenced by the privileged Greco-Roman tradition, or not. How much did theoretical medicine affect the way people were treated? Was there a large difference between the way the

1 During the Middle Ages, *physica* could adhere to its earlier meaning of natural philosophy, but was also used interchangeably with *medicina*, or medicine as practiced. Earlier and later writers, however, held the two meanings to be distinct from each other (Bylebyl 1990).

Vaughan, Theresa A., *Women, Food, and Diet in the Middle Ages: Balancing the Humours.* Taylor & Francis Group, 2020
DOI: 10.5117/9789462989382_CH04

different social classes sought medical care and the way those with money and prestige sought medical care?

Some of these questions are tackled by significant scholars on medicine and health in the Middle Ages, people like Monica Green, Bruno Laurioux, Madeleine Nicoud, Ken Albala, Faith Wallis and Melitta Weiss-Amer. While it's certainly possible to trace the textual tradition through the medieval West, and there is some surviving evidence of medicine as practiced, this evidence usually comes from the literate classes, and is therefore more likely to be in the theoretical tradition. This chapter summarizes some of that material (much of it already mentioned in Chapter Two and Chapter Three), and introduces some of the major works that deal with medicine in the Middle Ages, particularly as it pertained to the treatment of women.

It should also be noted that folk belief and folk religion can be intimately intertwined with medicine. We know, for example, in ancient Greece, that medicine and religious healing existed side by side (Siraisi 2009, 2). This is the norm in most societies. Sometimes medicine is more separated from religious healing, sometimes it is deeply related. When we look at traditional[2] medicine in the Middle Ages, we have several factors at play. First is theoretical medicine, for which we have an excellent record. Second, there is practical medicine, or empirically-based medicine, which may be more or less influenced by theoretical medicine. It may also be influenced by traditional or folk medicine. Third, you have traditional or folk medicine, terms I often use interchangeably in this text, though in this chapter make a distinction between them. Finally, there is religion; in medieval Europe, it may be the sanctioned medicine of the Catholic Church, or folk belief more or less related to pre-Christian practices and beliefs. This topic is explored further in Chapter Eight.

While we clearly have the best evidence for the literate tradition, I draw on, where possible, evidence for less privileged medicine, such as folk medicine and medicine practiced by women. As introduced in Chapter Three, folklore is present in the *Distaff Gospels*, and Garay and Jeay (2007) argue that the medical advice portrayed in that work is likely to be actual folk medicine as practiced by women in Picardie. I explore that in more depth, then suggest some other sources that may tell us something about folk medicine. Again, I focus on the treatment of women and women's health concerns.

Finally, what can be said about diet and health practices among common people, or advice as dispensed by lay medical practitioners, as well as how folk medicine, magic, and theoretical medicine might intertwine? By the

2 Defined more precisely later in this chapter.

time we get to the *Regimina sanitatis* of the 1300s and beyond, we know there were books available about diet for non-specialists. But then again, these texts were certainly in the hands of the literate, who tended to be either wealthy or part of the ecclesiastical tradition. It is difficult to make any definitive declarations about folk medicine, but we can speculate based on what evidence we do have, and what we know about folk medicine in general and in other cultures.

The medieval diet

The medieval diet relied on a number of factors. The diet of the common peasant or lower-class town dweller may have been based upon ideas of health, but was much more likely to be based on what was available and grown or produced locally. Local food traditions dictated what dishes were available for special feast days, but the normal day to day diet was largely made up of bread, wine or ale, cooked vegetables and herbs, and occasional meat, typically used as flavouring for pottage (Laurioux 2002). Did medieval people think of their daily diet at all in terms of health and disease, as practitioners of theoretical medicine most certainly did? Possibly not.

Another factor not yet addressed is the influence of the Church on the diet of both the poor and the wealthy. This effect would be two-fold. First, the complex series of feast days and fast days in the Church calendar dictated what one could eat on different days of the year. For the wealthy, fast day food could be made to look as much like feast day food as possible, with skilled cooks and Church-approved ingredients. For the common people, fast days meant dried or salted fish, bread without butter or oil, and pottage with only herbs to supply extra flavour (Lozinski 1933). An inconvenience for the wealthy might be a hardship for the poor, not just in terms of taste, but also of nutrition. Second, the Church taught that gluttony was a cardinal sin – that eating should be controlled, and one should consume just enough to maintain health. Overindulgence should be avoided, both in terms of quantity and quality of food, lest diet lead to the inflammation of the passions and temptation to further sin. Again, this could be ignored to an extent by the wealthy, if they chose, but for the peasant who experienced times of the year when it was impossible to overeat due to the seasonal scarcity of food[3], the Church's teachings might be a hardship.

3 This was especially true in late winter into spring, when the autumn harvest was mostly consumed, but new grains and plants, as well as milk or eggs, were not yet available.

Folk medicine

In contemporary terms, folk medicine is any medicine that is not allopathic – that is, not part of the Western medical model based upon classifications of disease and treatment, usually with surgery or pharmaceuticals. Actually, it's more complicated than that: there's traditional medicine, which may in itself have a long-established theoretical basis (such as Chinese Traditional Medicine or Ayurvedic Medicine), and which is usually administered by formally trained health practitioners. To a degree, the theoretical Western tradition can be viewed this way. Holistic medicine – which has become popular in the West – seeks to treat the whole person, not just the disease. Disease-focused treatment is one of the hallmarks of Western allopathic medicine. It tends to draw somewhat eclectically from numerous established traditions, plus more modern developments – like biofeedback, for example – but retains a firm basis in Western allopathic medicine. Folk medicine itself often has a holistic orientation. There's alternative medicine, which again may draw from many established traditions, but which often eschews allopathic medicine. Alternative medicine might involve radical changes to diet and herbal remedies or homeopathy to create a healthy environment for the body and treat disease by 'natural' means. The term 'natural' is itself problematic, but that's how it is normally defined. There are traditional medicines also sometimes called folk medicine – such as those of indigenous peoples – that typically share a spiritual component along with indigenous theories of illness and wholeness.

As previously noted, theoretical medicine in the Middle Ages did involve the use of herbs, just as folk medicine, but beginning in the nineteenth-century, theoretical medicine began moving away from herbs as knowledge of chemistry progressed and the focus switched to isolate medicinal compounds, using them in isolation and in stronger concentration. Folk medicine itself is often seen as medicine learned informally. It is passed down orally, and includes treatments which may be based on herbal remedies, conforming to the doctrine of signatures or other folk theories of healing (Bennett 2007)[4]. This type of medicine, as studied by anthropologists and folklorists, is most common today among immigrant communities, rural dwellers, and people who live traditionally (Brady 2001). It is medicine passed down in families, often by women, existing outside the realm of formal medical education and practice.

4 There is some debate about whether or not, using the doctrine of signatures, plants are identified first using their resemblance to some part of the body, or whether that resemblance is considered post-hoc, and is simply used as a mnemonic device in orally-transmitted medicine.

Folk medicine is a complex system of medical beliefs, which the contemporary West sometimes frowns upon – allopathic medicine, after all, has the backing of hard science. Folk medicine in this context can sometimes refer to any medicine that is not allopathic. That view is too simplistic to make much of a contribution to the understanding of the medical landscape. Often, people who avail themselves of allopathic medicine, but come from a background in which other forms of medicine are used – traditional or folk medicine – don't report their pursuit of other treatments to their doctors, fearing condemnation or being treated as ignorant by a physician. Sometimes this can interfere with allopathic treatment involving pharmaceuticals, as some traditional medicine can cross-react with contemporary drugs. There is a body of literature in medicine that seeks to explain and sometimes incorporate better understanding of these alternative modes of healing into Western medicine. But much disdain exists in the medical community for some alternative forms of treatment; witness the continuing debate over 'supplements' or 'nutraceuticals' playing out in the news. Supplements, however, are somewhat outside the realm of folk medicine because they commercialize folk remedies or rely on an appeal to 'natural' remedies for mass market purposes. There are disagreements on the science behind supplements, and concern about the purity and efficacy of mass-produced supplements. Supplements and miracle cures, often loosely tied to indigenous folk medicine, can inspire false claims, as well as rumour and legend on the internet (Kitta 2018).

Medieval medicine and folk medicine

The world of medieval medicine was no less complex, though some of the arguments and types of practitioners were framed differently. There were several classifications of healers, each with their own characteristic treatments, training, and responsibilities. Which kind of healer one consulted depended upon social class and whether one lived in the city, town, or countryside, where the availability of different kinds of practitioners was lacking. Those who were academically trained were considered *doctor medicinae*, those who earned a university degree. These medical practitioners were the most familiar with theoretical medicine, as it was integral to their training. There was also the surgeon, one formally trained in anatomy and the art of surgery. Some schools of medicine, once established, taught surgery to medical students, while in other areas the practices remained separate. In many cases, surgery was considered a craft, rather than an art, and so was of somewhat lower status. Below the surgeon in the level of training received was the barber-surgeon. The barber-surgeon would have had very sharp knives and was in demand as a barber – for monk's tonsures as well as other cutting and shaving – but might also practice basic dentistry and blood-letting. Most famously, barber-surgeons were needed during times of war, where they were available for amputations and other battlefield medical procedures. Priests and monks might have been familiar with basic medicine, and could, of course, also apply spiritual treatments for disease. Apothecaries were trained in the practice of measuring and dispensing medicines and spices, and also provided general medical advice. Wise-women and midwives were female medical practitioners who dealt with a number of medical problems. They would of course help with the birth process, but were also familiar with herbal remedies and traditional methods of healing, the closest to what would be considered folk medicine today. Empirically-grounded 'leeches'[5], or lay medical practitioners empirically rather than theoretically trained, formed another tier of those available to medieval people. Finally, within a family, a person, often a mother, might take on the task of treating minor complaints or bandaging wounds (Stannard 2013, 47).

Medicine of the medieval period was based on diet, as we have seen, and on simples, natural products of plant, animal, or mineral origin. Plants formed the largest group of these simples. Thus, herbal medicine formed the largest category of medicine in medieval Europe. Some of the medicinal preparations were quite complex, involving multiple steps of processing and many different ingredients. While this book focuses on diet in the treatment of disease and promotion of health for women, we cannot ignore the importance of medical preparations from natural ingredients. Of course, one great difference with the present day is that most drugs are now synthetically produced, rather than relying upon plants, animals, or minerals. Here, the legacy of folk medicine can be placed largely among those who were not the product of theoretical medical training, but the informal training that occurred within families, or through apprenticeship and observation of other practitioners. These would have been the point of contact for most medieval people of modest means – wise women, midwives, leeches, and barber-surgeons (Stannard 2013).

Evidence for medieval medicine based largely upon plant-based remedies can be found in three different types of written sources, though much may have been transmitted orally. First is the *receptarium*, loosely translated as a 'recipe collection'. These *receptaria* have been found in

5 This term was used in England, but there were equivalent categories in other areas.

many different lengths, literary styles, and competencies. The primary purpose of a *receptarium* was to record information both for practice and for posterity. In the majority of cases, each recipe included four different elements: 'purpose, enumeration of the ingredients, method of preparation, and mode of administration' (Stannard 2013, 49).

A second genre of medieval medical literature is the herbal. An herbal consists of a list of plants, their properties, and their uses. The herbal systematizes knowledge of plants and their medical properties. Unlike the *receptarium*, where recipes were arranged by ailment (or not at all), the herbal was an organized way of conveying botanical information. Some herbals were considered highly valuable in medieval and early modern medicine, and had antecedents in antiquity (Everett 2014). Herbals continued to be the primary way of communicating botanical information until the seventeenth century.

A third type of medical genre that developed during the course of the Middle Ages is known as the *leechbook*. Leechbooks were general guides to health and all-purpose medical manuals highly variable in nature. They contained a great variety of material, including recipes and miniature herbals. They were formatted to accommodate new material and information over time (Stannard 2013, 49).

Thus, medicinal properties of plants were known and transmitted. At the same time, information was also being passed down orally in the province of folk medicine. The primary diseases and treatments were probably known to both professionals and to many lay medical practitioners (Stannard 2013; Quave, Pardo-de-Santayana, and Pieroni 2012). We can use some surviving folk knowledge to guess at what might have been part of the oral medical tradition of the Middle Ages. Of course, however, some of that information would be similar, some will have disappeared, and some has been added since that time. This is why documents such as the *Distaff Gospels*, which offer oral lore that includes some folk medicine, are so important (Jeay 1982).

Stannard (2012) suggests that there were at least a certain number of plant species whose properties were common knowledge, and which likely played a role in medieval folk medicine as well as theoretical medicine. Some were used primarily as common foodstuffs, such as wheat and barley, cabbage, apples, quinces, and certain nuts. However, all of these could also function as a medicine, depending upon preparation. Some could become part of medicinal preparations that contained other substances, known as *composita*. There were also many herbs with widely- known properties, recognizable to most people. There are about thirty of these most common species, and they include sage, dill, rue, hyssop, marjoram, parsley, and garlic. While herbals and other medical texts might mention hundreds of plants and their properties, these very commonly known herbs were likely components of folk medicine. In fact, many of these primary herbs are still included in European folk medicine today, and are also integral parts of regional and national cuisines, a legacy, perhaps, of food as medicine, and serving as herbal flavourings to make the taste of relatively bland grains more appealing. These common herbs were available to everyone if they grew in the region, and were not prohibitively expensive, such as more exotic spices.

Women and folk medicine

Women were more likely to be limited to the practice of practical or folk medicine. Barred from becoming university-educated physicians for most of the Middle Ages, women were not completely shut out of practicing medicine of some kind. Monica Green argues it is likely that women did act as medical practitioners, though in categories less likely to be officially noticed or recorded. There are three categories in which women were likely to be placed as healers: first, as *vetulae*. The term itself means 'old woman', and was attached to women healers deemed illiterate, ignorant, superstitious, too rural, or too old to actually know anything (Green 2000c, 336). In modern vernacular English, the term 'old wives' tale' for a folk belief with no basis in fact, uses the same disparaging tone toward older women and their wisdom. The term may have been used by physicians to actively disparage women who were traditional healers. The fact that the word seems to have been in wide use most likely indicates that there were a significant number of women who did act as traditional healers.

The second category of (largely) female healers was midwives. While an increasing amount of academic work on midwives has been done, it is often difficult to get a clear idea of exactly how they practiced, their knowledge, and their reputations. While we know that midwives were sometimes associated with ignorance, greed, and unsavoury practices, they could also be respected medical practitioners, whose services might even be used by royalty (Mormiche and Perez 2016). Green (2000c) notes that the relative lack of documentation of midwives might be due to the fact that they were not members of guilds, nor had they any formal affiliation with medical schools or hospitals. They were not officially licensed until the fifteenth century. Places where they may have been more frequently mentioned, such as in parish records, still remain relatively unexamined (Green 2000c,

338). We have visual evidence of midwives, such as in scenes of the nativity or royal births, but these are usually set pieces that take place after birth, when the woman is clean and the baby is being bathed or swaddled; they don't give much information about what midwives actually did (Berthiaud 2016). In fact, women who were referred to as *vetulae* may have served as midwives, since evidence suggests that the knowledge of basic midwifery may have been common among many women (Green 2000c).

Nurse is another problematic category, in that our modern understanding of a nurse's work is influenced by professional nursing as it has existed since the nineteenth century. Before that point, the term nurse might represent a wet-nurse, a nanny, a woman religious (nun), hospital attendant, or many other kinds of caretakers.

It is probably fair to say that women were limited mostly to practical or traditional medicine, with, of course, some exceptions. Some women served as physicians (most likely trained by their husbands) and barber-surgeons. They usually appear in a significantly small minority of the healing professions for which records were kept, though, again, records were not kept for a number of medical specialities, such as midwifery, until late in the Middle Ages (Green 2000c). Among medical practitioners for whom official records do exist – physicians, apothecaries, and barber-surgeons, for example – women seem to have treated both men and women.

We can say that women did sometimes practice medicine formally, and would have perhaps been familiar with some theoretical medicine. More often, however, those with knowledge of folk or traditional medicine were actively denigrated. Women were not, of course, the sole repository of traditional medicine; some men must have been as well. We can see them mocked in the profession of barber, or sometimes associated with magic or questionable forms of healing frowned upon by the Church. But it seems women did have a prominent role in the passing on of traditional medical knowledge.

Theoretical medicine and folk medicine

The distinction between theoretical and folk medicine seems clear: one being professionalized, largely male, and based upon a theoretical tradition that derived from antiquity; the other based on traditional knowledge, informally passed through the oral tradition, being at least overtly divorced from theoretical medicine, and demonstrating some of the typical hallmarks of folk medicine, such as the use of the doctrine of signatures and reliance on sympathetic magic. What then shall we do about what is called in the literature 'practical medicine'? If we place folk medicine and theoretical medicine at opposite ends of a continuum, practical medicine might fall between the two. Practical medicine is empirically-based, meaning it is based on what has been tried and proven effective often enough that it continues to be done, rather than specifically based upon theory or traditions coming from the 'folk'. Folk medicine can also be theoretical, based on folk or indigenous understanding of the body and disease. Practical medicine can, of course, have treatments and practices that come from either folk medicine or the theoretical medical tradition, but is grounded in practice and successful treatment.

As medicine grows more and more professionalized starting in the thirteenth century, it becomes more difficult to assess women's voices in medicine. 'As theoretical learning came to be increasingly valued in the legal assessment of the curative merits of healers, would it not be inevitable that women's capabilities be increasingly devalued since they had so little access to that learning? The common belief in women's feeble intellectual abilities could only have enhanced prejudices against them further' (Green 2000c, 350).

Historians writing about medieval medicine typically speak about theoretical vs. practical medicine, rather than including folk medicine explicitly, perhaps because theoretical medicine, and some practical medicine, is certainly easier to get at than folk medicine. Practical medicine may also be seen as stemming in part from theoretical medicine. But folk medicine is a useful category to add to the mix, because it might help us understand how medicine worked among those not wealthy enough to afford the services of a university-trained physician, nor necessarily even that of practical medicus or barber. It is also the category where, I assert, we are most likely to find women as practitioners.

By the fifteenth and sixteenth centuries, it was increasingly likely that a woman who practiced folk medicine or theoretical medicine without being university-trained, would be associated with witchcraft. Since illness itself was often understood to be the result of sin within the Western Christian worldview, women who operated as medical practitioners outside the realm of respected practical or theoretical medicine might be in league with the devil in curing diseases, or delivering babies with the sole aim of using the infants for nefarious purposes. While the high point of accusations and trials for witchcraft occurred from the later fifteenth through the seventeenth centuries, elements of this prejudice and fear of peasant women became increasingly evident (Smith 2007b).

According to some writers, the connection of women healers with witchcraft came about as medicine professionalized, and rustic women healers were seen either as charlatans, or as gaining power to heal or inflict injury as a result of a pact made with the devil:

> Many peasant healers believed that admitted witches possessed the skills of sorcery, a widely held view of the witch, and they denied holding membership in the occult sorority and applying witchcraft to their healing practices (Minkowsky 1992, 294).

There is some debate over whether midwives were particularly targeted for witchcraft accusations. David Harley asserts that, while women medical practitioners could be the target of witchcraft allegations in the Early Modern period, midwives themselves were rarely accused, unless there were some particular local belief to prompt such concerns. However, studies do indicate that women healers were particularly subject to witchcraft allegations, as well as those trades associated with food preparation or magical medicine (Harley 1990). The connection of midwives with witchcraft, such as that noted above by Minkowski, could be a result of a misinterpretation of the records or an overly hasty analysis by some early scholars.

The therapies these women employed were usually derived from folk medicine and folk belief, always deemed suspicious by the Church. Their low social status and often their poverty left them vulnerable to accusations without the power to refute them. Some perhaps did undertake to learn and practice what was understood to be magic and witchcraft at the time period, to make their work more efficacious, or to pull themselves out of poverty and make life better for themselves or their families (Minkowsky 1992). We can see in pseudo-Albertus' *De secretis mulierum,* mentioned previously, the association of women with imperfection, poison, degradation, and stupidity, along with wiliness, evil, and selfishness (Lemay 1992); from here, it's not unreasonable for the monks and more powerful church figures to see women practitioners as somehow in league with the devil. The fifteenth century *Distaff Gospels* contains evidence that, at least in the popular imagination of the aristocracy, women who practiced healing were also associated with heresy and witchcraft (Garay and Jeay 2007). 'By the late Middle Ages, the church and civil authorities mandated close supervision of midwives, as expressed in required professional and religious instruction and in oaths that explicitly renounced past and present resort to the black arts' (Minkowsky 1992, 294).

As we can see above, the Church came to associate at least some kinds of folk medicine with tampering with the supernatural. We can narrow the distinction by classifying who practiced the medicine: perhaps folk medicine itself was simply practiced by the peasant, by the illiterate. Does that mean it was only belief-based, and not empirical?

At what point does it become meaningful to distinguish between academic medicine and folk medicine in the Middle Ages? Certainly medieval people, or at least academically-trained doctors, viewed them as different to some meaningful extent. Are they both merely constructs of ways of understanding illness and the body, and thus should be treated the same way? We can recognize the different foundations of these two types of medicine, but also see they share the same aims – the promotion of good health and the treatment of disease.

The ways folklorists talk about folk versus professional medicine often do not align with the approaches of historians. How do we make a distinction between folk medicine, learned or professional medicine, and magic during the medieval era from an interdisciplinary point of view? In part by making a distinction between medieval and contemporary understandings of medical efficacy and the underpinnings of magic and folk medicine.

Folklorists O'Connor and Hufford (2001) have outlined several characteristics of folk medicine. They emphasize the mode of transmission (informal or oral) and the relative status of the medical system (generally low, at least in countries that privilege allopathic modalities). They also mention that folk understandings of bodily health focus on balance and harmony. Another characteristic we see today in the way the professional medical community regards folk medicine is the use of herbs and natural substances in the healing process and in the making of medicaments. In looking back at the Middle Ages, however, we cannot solely point to the use of herbal medicine for evidence of folk medicine, for herbs and plants were used by university trained physicians as well as by the 'old wives' (Gentilcore 2004). We can point to folk medicine as that which was learned informally, through apprenticeship and imitative use, rather than through books or formal schools. However, before the thirteenth century, many doctors learned practical medicine through apprenticeship and practice, as well as midwives or wise women. The only consistent difference is status, but even that was fluid particularly between the fourth and twelfth centuries, before the advent of medical schools.

Before the establishment of medical schools, the medicine practiced in monasteries was given the highest status. Monasteries were the repositories of medical manuscripts, and also served as locations where the community

Domestic Judicial Treatment of European Court of Human Rights Case Law

Beyond Compliance

David Kosař, Jan Petrov, Katarína Šipulová, Hubert Smekal, Ladislav Vyhnánek, and Jozef Janovský

Routledge
Taylor & Francis Group
LONDON AND NEW YORK

could obtain treatment. The manuscripts were those of the Greek medical tradition, although the Church also introduced a degree of suspicion for 'pagan' medicine in the early medieval period. What bearing does this have on folk medicine? Although the term 'folk' may have an uneasy relationship with the common people of the Middle Ages – after all, the word was initially applied to European peasants of the eighteenth and nineteenth centuries – can it be applied to the majority of medieval people? Perhaps medieval folk medicine itself was simply medicine practiced by the peasant, by the illiterate. Historians often use the term 'popular medicine' rather than 'folk medicine', referring to the general populace rather than the aristocracy or Church community. But does being of the folk, or of the common people, mean medicine lacked empirical characteristics?

One of the ironies of the distinction between folk and professional medicine in the Middle Ages is that what historians now view as learned or professional medicine – the inheritance of the written Hippocratic and Galenic as practiced by literate and, after the twelfth century, university trained physicians – is now considered folk medicine. Vestiges of Greco-Roman humoral theory still survive in the classification of foodstuffs as 'hot' and 'cold' by some who practice folk medicine (Hand 1976, 4). The emphasis on 'balance' in the humoral system – the idea that imbalance in the humours caused illness – is also now considered part of folk medicine, even if the humours are not referred to directly. Many examples of European folk medicine include ideas traced back through the Middle Ages to the ancient world (Talbot 1976). Tracking specific beliefs farther than the 1800s is sometimes difficult, although that again relies upon written sources (Retief and Cilliers 2001).

This brings us back to the practice of professional versus folk medicine in the Middle Ages. There are differences between the way historians have written about 'practical' or 'folk' medicine and the ways in which folklorists or anthropologists address it. Greek medical tradition privileges medicine as it derives from natural philosophy. However, there is also evidence for medical treatments not derived from the ideas of natural philosophy. We know, for example, that Hippocrates, Soranus, and Galen were all practicing physicians. Their understanding of medicine was grounded partially in the philosophical tradition, but they also drew from empirical knowledge in their treatment of patients and their variety of ailments. Their recommendations also draw, in a minor way, from local knowledge: foods considered appropriate for the invalid were local staples. Hippocrates, for example, thought especially highly of the recuperative powers of barley, a common grain in his region.

Efficacy and folk belief

As far back as the writers of the Hippocratic Corpus, there was a distrust of medicine based upon what writers termed 'superstition', as opposed to the (supposedly) rational medicine of the Greco-Roman tradition. Radical changes in understanding bodily functions and the transmission of disease eventually overturned the Greco-Roman foundation of European medicine, but it would take until the mid-eighteenth century for this to appear in the written tradition, albeit longer in practice.

Can a distinction between types of medicine be made in terms of perceived effectiveness? How did medieval people judge the effectiveness of learned medicine, and did they judge folk medicine any differently? Medieval Christianity sometimes coexisted uneasily with the written medical tradition, and medieval medical writers are generally clear that their recommendations would only work if God willed them so, and that God could cure a patient even when medicine could not (Retief and Cilliers 2001). The Church was also generally leery of 'magic', which they understood to be supernatural forces outside the realm of those sanctioned by orthodox belief to effect healing.

Stanley J. Tambiah argues that the effectiveness of magic, and by extension, the effectiveness of medieval medicine, was judged wholly differently from the contemporary scientific worldview. In the Middle Ages, the principles employed in magic, such as the principle of like influences like (sympathetic magic), are also clearly present in both pharmacological and dietary treatment of illness (Tambiah 2017 [1973]).

Tambiah, an anthropologist who spent his years as a professor at Harvard University, was born and received his early education in Sri Lanka. As a non-Western man trained largely in the Western anthropological tradition, he brought to bear both emic and etic[6] points of view on his subject matter. In 'Form and Meaning of Magical Acts', an article serving as a precursor to his longer monograph *Magic, Science, Religion, and the Scope of Rationality,* Tambiah (2017 [1973]) argues that using the Western, post-Enlightenment view of scientific cause and effect to judge the effectiveness of what Westerners view as nonsensical causative acts in other cultures (magic), is not a

6 An 'emic' view considers worldview from the point of view of an insider, one with long-term intimate familiarity with a culture. An 'etic' view is the point of view of an outsider, or one who may be familiar with a culture, but not as a member of that culture. In anthropological work, it can be described as the switch from analyzing a culture from the perspective of a member of that culture (subjective), to describing a culture from the frame of the anthropologist (objective). The two terms come ultimately from the differentiation in linguistics between phonemic (sound as spoken) and phonetic (sound as described).

useful way of understanding how to observe those acts. Magic, according to Tambiah, is not subject to the same set of causal relationships as Western science. Things are not as simple as 'mystical' vs 'empirical', for as discussed earlier, these concepts blurred into one another.

Magical acts, says Tambiah, typically involve a verbal utterance plus object manipulation. They are, in fact, performative acts. In addition, magical acts can be viewed as ritual acts, and ritual acts as performative acts not subject to empirical verification. It is the act itself that is important, rather than the specifics of the outcome. Science, on the other hand, makes the known stand as a model for the incompletely known. That model suggests a prediction, and is then subject to empirical tests: observation and verification to ascertain the truth value. The ultimate difference here is that with magic, as with ritual, the act itself is important rather than the verifiable outcome. By contemporary standards, both learned and informal medicine appear to be ineffective in most cases, but medieval people, if we follow Tambiah, would not have judged them in the same way, because they existed before Enlightenment models of scientific inquiry.

What does this have to do with the difference between medieval folk medicine, professional medicine, and the medicine of today? Soranus describes the ideal midwife as a woman who is not superstitious, but empirical. She must be trained in the rational tradition, and not resort to charms or other forms of what we might call folk belief. While not operating in terms of contemporary understanding of science, Soranus clearly drew a line between professional medicine and what he termed 'superstition', which he clearly associates with women's traditional knowledge. Medieval medical schools emphasized the importance of theoretical medicine based upon the ancient writers (as all Greek and Roman written work was privileged) as fundamentally different from superstition and suspect medicine, especially that practiced informally by women.

In fact, if we look at both herbal medicines and dietary recommendations from the Middle Ages, we can see evidence of the pre-Enlightenment, and in a sense, pre-scientific worldview examined by Tambiah. Humoral theory is considered provably false by contemporary standards of medicine. Many medieval medicines, though not all, also fail the test of empirical verification. In fact, the efficacy of certain herbal medicines was based entirely on ideas of sympathetic magic (like influences like) or what Paracelsus would call (Theophrastus von Hohenheim, 1493-1541 CE, Einsiedeln, Switzerland) the 'doctrine of signatures' (Pearce 2008).

Can these remedies be considered scientific in the modern sense? The answer is that, by and large, they can't. The medieval textual tradition of theoretical medicine was built up by people quoting both ancient and more contemporary authors, sometimes with attribution and sometimes not, often in a haphazard way: adding their own ideas (while sometimes identifying them as the ideas of someone more ancient to lend them more credence) as they went along. 'Empirical' medicine coexisted with the theoretical in the written tradition – techniques for dealing with difficult births, general recommendations for health involving exercise and moderation (and there is some evidence that physicians used herbs, compounded medicine, and suggested diets because they believed them to be efficacious) – but this idea of efficacy seems to have been largely built on the theoretical tradition. How are these ideas related to the efficacy of magic as posited by Tambiah?

Women as healers

The subject of magic in the Middle Ages is immense, so let us confine ourselves here to a narrower focus: healing done by women. This is not to say that men were not capable or accused of using magic, but in the realm of medicine and folk belief, women were typically the keepers of the household traditions of healing on a daily basis passed along orally. This is what ancient and medieval writers derided as 'superstition' or appealing to knowledge and forces outside what was sanctioned by the Church (who eventually supported the Galenic tradition and condemned as heresy any medical understanding outside of that tradition). We can see evidence of this in a number of sources, but let us take as an example the *Distaff Gospels,* previously described. There is good evidence that many of the 'gospels' reported here are recorded instances of local folklore, told by women and presented here as the amusing speech of older women – in short, old wives' tales. The women who proclaim their gospels each night are themselves a motley collection of heretics, prostitutes, women practicing medicine illegally, and other amusing characters. Still, the recorded folklore is likely to be accurate for Flanders and Picardie of the time (Jeay 1982).

Mixed with fantasies of what women do to cheating or violent husbands, we see both magic and medicine. One of the women who meets to proclaim her gospel is 'Berthe de Corne', a woman whose father was a doctor trained in the medical school of Montpellier, and who passed on some of his knowledge to her. It is implied that she practices medicine, although this was illegal for women. Her gospels adhere more closely to the language of the written medical tradition than do those of other women, and she gives remedies for various kinds of fevers (quartan, tertian, continuous), measles, and smallpox. Her remedies, however, fall more along the lines of folk medicine and religious magic. For example, a woman with measles should take holy water, prepare a broth with it, and then drink it; she would then be cured (Garay and Jeay 2006, 177).

Other women do not use such technical medical language, tending to make pronouncements about how to avoid illness or misfortune, rather than cure it. Interestingly, a number of the beliefs reported in the *Distaff Gospels* still exist in some form today. Paul Sébillot compiled a list of folk beliefs and practices in a multi-volume set published from the late 1800s to the early 1900s called *Le folk-lore de France*. These instances of folklore were collected in approximately the same area of France where the *Distaff Gospels* were written, and there are some striking parallels. Even farther afield, similar beliefs can be found in the Fife Collection at Utah State University (1976, 278)[7], which catalogues folk medicine and beliefs collected in the United States. However, one can also find mention of this same belief in the medical texts, such as in the *Trotula*.

There are a few specific cures, but they tend to be for ridding oneself of warts or headaches, common household concerns that would not merit consulting a healer. There are many folk remedies to cure warts. In the *Distaff Gospels,* the recommendation is to rub the wart with the leaf of an elder tree on Midsummer's Even, then bury the leaf. After it has decomposed, the wart will fall off (Garay and Jeay 2006, 213). This is an example of how women were responsible for routine healing, relying primarily on traditional practices passed down orally, rather than as a part of the written tradition.

Magic and belief

The line between magic and folk practices of divination and methods of controlling the environment is essentially non-existent in this text. That was part of the humour of the manuscript: that these old women dabbled both

7 The use of the American Fife Collection is not unrelated to an examination of European folk medicine. It is likely that some traces of medieval medicine came with European settlers, and are thus found in American folk medicine (Hand 1976, 4). It is also the case that traces of medieval medical beliefs are present in European folk medicine today. We find contemporary beliefs in 'mad stones', which are really just the bezoars (naturally occurring concretions of the digestive tract thought to provide an antidote to certain ailments) of the Middle Ages (Forbes 1976) and the use of certain plants as medicine for certain ailments, such as the peony for epilepsy (Talbot 1976). These beliefs vary from the medical theories and healing modalities of indigenous Americans and are thus of European origin.

with practicing medicine illegally and unsanctioned supernatural forces. It is here that Tambiah's understanding is relevant if we wish to understand the 'effectiveness' of these prescriptions. In each one, a performative act is described by the woman in order to obtain a certain outcome, such as the instructions for ridding oneself of a wart or curing a headache. If performative acts are ritual acts, then their effectiveness is not necessarily subject to empirical verification. Part of what the women in the *Distaff Gospels* swear, however, in a rather formulaic way, are that these acts are efficacious – or are up to a point. Does that negate what Tambiah indicates with respect to magic? No, because these are instances of folklore set within a conventional narrative frame: the audience expects that the clerk recording these instances will emphasize that these ridiculous old women actually believe what they say and will swear to it, while he himself belittles them for their superstitious and magical practices. He is of a higher class, as part of the learned written tradition (as literacy was the fundamental requirement of a clerk), so it would be absurd for him to promote these beliefs. These are old wives' tales, after all. The idea of making fun of the credulity of the unlearned was part of elite culture (Gates 1997), and this is, at its root, the source of humour in the text.

When we compare this example to the healing attributed to doctors, especially university-trained physicians as they began to appear in the twelfth century and later, we can see that doctors had at their disposal a textual tradition from which to draw. This tradition, because it is textual, had the aura of authority that folk medicine does not. In the medieval period, this elite status would distinguish it from folk medicine, even if it was based upon balance, and even if its own efficacy as we now understand it was similarly poor.

An exception to this may be herbal medicine as it was passed down orally. But even there, the idea of sympathetic magic may be more apparent, though it is certainly not absent in the case of the medical textual tradition; in fact, it is fundamental to the use of some plants in the making of medicines. How then do we judge the efficacy of medical treatments, and do they still relate to Tambiah's statements about ritual efficacy? They have the veneer of legitimacy, though it is clear by contemporary standards of measuring treatment efficacy that many, if not most, of these treatments were really based upon the ritual of treatment, rather than some contemporary notion of science and provability. The veneer of authority given to textual medical traditions and to university physicians was a matter of social circumstance rather than a contemporary understanding of science or the efficacy of treatment. Folk medicine, or medicine as it was practiced by women, did not have that authority. Does some folk medicine 'work' in the modern sense? Possibly. Did some medicine of the text-based tradition work? Possibly as well. In both cases, the treatment or remedy was based on some authority: in the case of folk medicine, the authority of tradition[8]; in the case of learned medicine, the authority of written texts and, it must be said, tradition as well.

The manuscripts described here do relate to the intellectual traditions of Western culture, with some ideas about rational thought coming from the ancient Greeks. The Greco-Roman writers built a foundation on which the medieval writers constructed their understanding of a 'scientific' medicine. While a number of influences modified the Greco-Roman tradition over time, both in terms of understanding the body and in developing new medical techniques through both experience and the incorporation of local and foreign traditions, the sea change that influenced the medieval worldview was, of course, Christianity. While this topic is explored more fully in Chapter Eight, a few pertinent points will help when considering the following chapters.

As we will see most explicitly with the writings of Hildegard of Bingen in Chapter Five, a Christian view of healing was not dismissive of the Greco-Roman medical tradition by the eleventh century, but assumed that God's will superseded any medical treatment. A healer could do his or her best, but if healing was not God's will, the patient would not improve. Likewise, the invocation of Jesus, Mary, or the saints during illness could be seen as adding efficacy to the healing efforts. If we look at childbirth, for example, the textual tradition discusses how to deal with birth problems, but, in addition, especially by the later part of the Middle Ages, prayers were said, holy girdles were worn, amulets were produced, and other largely religious measures were taken to help ensure a positive outcome. These might be used alongside measures that we now consider 'superstition', or part of the folk belief at the time: the use of bezoars, charms, and other strategies for invoking non-medical powers in the act of healing. The average person would not see any incompatibility between religion, professional medicine, folk medicine, and folk belief. Of course, the Church frowned upon the use of anything considered unduly 'magical', in the sense that it may have come from evil or demonic forces. But we must remember, the view of what constituted magic differed in the medieval world.

8 The definition and characteristics of 'tradition' are the subject of debate in both folklore and anthropology. The fields have moved from thinking of traditions as survivals from some ancient past to cultural practices that are dynamic and changing, though with some sense of conservation. Traditions can be invented, modified, or carried forward because they still have a function within a culture (Glassie 1995).

5 The *Trotula* and the Works of Hildegard of Bingen

Abstract
Two thirteenth century works on medicine attributed to women are examined for what they tell us about those writing inside and outside the medical tradition, and what the authors might have known about folk medicine. The *Trotula* is traditionally attributed to a female author (Trota) who was a teacher in the medical school at Salerno. While only part of the book, if any, was written by Trota, the text was a mainstay of gynaecological treatment through the sixteenth century. Hildegard of Bingen was a prolific author and abbess who wrote two works addressing health: *Causae et curae* and *Physica*. All three texts are examined and compared for their take on humoral theory and influence of folk medicine.

Keywords: *Trotula*, Hildegard of Bingen, humoral theory, gynaecology, dietetics, folk medicine

In this chapter, I look more closely at three works attributed to women writing in the twelfth century. One work, the *Trotula*, was probably not written by a woman, at least not in its entirety. It was set firmly in the written theoretical tradition of Galen, and was copied and disseminated in various forms throughout the sixteenth century. The others are attributed to and most likely written by an abbess named Hildegard of Bingen. Her works are less firmly rooted in the Greek theoretical tradition, instead being a combination of her own view of natural philosophy and medicine informed by her own take on Christian theology. Each of these works are examined for their comments on food and diet for women, with an eye towards discovering what can be determined about their relationship to folk medicine and regional variation in food consumption patterns in terms of their treatment recommendations.

These two authors, Trota and Hildegard, might seem an odd choice for comparison, simply because there is a well-documented history of the

Vaughan, Theresa A., *Women, Food, and Diet in the Middle Ages: Balancing the Humours.* Taylor & Francis Group, 2020
DOI: 10.5117/9789462989382_CH05

works attributed to Trota being used extensively in the Western written medical tradition, while the same is not true of Hildegard. I have chosen the *Trotula* here specifically because it is one of the most accessible and widely used gynaecological texts of the time period. In searching for evidence of dietary recommendations for women's health in the medical tradition, this is a likely candidate. While there were general differences between the humoral makeup of men and women in medical texts, it is really only in works on gynaecology that we see women addressed specifically in any detail. In addition, the tradition that the *Trotula* was written by a woman was culturally significant, even if largely mistaken. The fact that medicine written about women was believed to be written by a woman says something about the hidden or secret nature of women's bodies in the larger culture – a woman was more likely than a man to know and understand these hidden things, or at least would be more easily privy to women's bodies. In addition, unlike some texts that are overtly hostile to women's bodies, the *Trotula* is more neutral and matter-of-fact in tone.

As for the works of Hildegard dealing with medicine and natural philosophy, why choose them if they were not really part of the longer written tradition? In part because this gives us a snapshot of a particular period in time, one in which we can compare and contrast perspectives on local and regional food, knowledge of herbs, and see how Church teachings may have influenced medicine in the monastic tradition. Hildegard's works were in fact written by a woman, and to some extent that is reflected in the writing itself. We can set these works within the corpus of an author whose biography is quite well known.

Both the *Trotula* and the works of Hildegard came out of the written tradition, but also out of the informal background of folk or popular medicine. In the *Trotula,* this is seen most clearly in that portion most likely to have been written by a female practicing physician. Both are theoretical in nature but contain practical advice for healing. Neither is divorced from the cultural context in which it was created. Even today, while a scientific orientation is supposed to be, ideally, culture-neutral, we can readily see the impact of different cultural orientations on how medicine is practiced and the theories chosen to explain the functioning of the body.

In the twelfth century, the population of Salerno was a mix of Christian, Muslim, and Jewish inhabitants. Being a port city, some direct trade brought the Salernitan population regular contact with other Mediterranean cities, but perhaps even more influential was Salerno's proximity to Sicily with its very active mixture of different cultures. The cross-cultural exchange of medical writings and ideas (Waines, 1999) was key to the development of medicine in Salerno. A 'school' of medicine had existed there for several centuries, and there were Salernitan medical treatises from before the twelfth century, most notably the *Regimen sanitatis Salerni*, compiled around 900 CE (Bifulco, Marasco, and Pisanti 2008). It was perhaps the most ancient school of medical knowledge in medieval Europe, predating the rise of the university. In addition, Salerno was the first European site of medical learning to take the more theoretical turn that would characterize medical training at universities (Wallis 2010, 129).

The *Trotula* emerges from a fruitful mix of traditions and cultures. Its three treatises were traditionally attributed to a single author, a female physician by the name of Trota associated with the Salernitan school of medicine. The treatises include: *Liber de sinthomatibus mulierum* or *Book on the Conditions of Women*; *De curis mulierum* or *On Treatments for Women*; and *De ornatu mulierum* or *On Women's Cosmetics*. While the actual authors are unknown, Green argues convincingly that *On Treatments for Women* was likely based upon the work of a practicing physician, perhaps the legendary Trota. As mentioned previously, this treatise may have been her own writing or a record of her teaching (Green 2002, 49-50). The entire collection concerns itself almost exclusively with women's health, with *Women's Cosmetics* comprised of head to toe beauty treatments, some based upon diet.[1]

Dietary recommendations in the collection are not numerous, comprising only seven of 131 entries in *Conditions of Women* and three of 110 entries in *Treatments for Women*. Herbs are frequently used for treatment either alone or in combination with other substances to make medicines. Sometimes wine, bacon fat, and other comestibles are used to process herbs or make them palatable, but those are not the focus of this analysis. Instead, we'll look at dietary recommendations.

From *Book on the Conditions of Women*

Book on the Conditions of Women begins with an initial description of the basic humoral qualities of men and women with reference to the works of Hippocrates and Galen. This treatise, one of the three forming the body of the *Trotula*, is the one most closely related to the tradition of Greco-Roman theoretical medicine. The description of women, based firmly in humoral

1 For an interesting contemporary reading of *On Women's Cosmetics*, see (Cavallo, Proto, Patruno, and Bifulco, 2008), written by faculty at the Department of Pharmaceutical Sciences at the University of Salerno.

theory, establishes the primary difference between men and women in humoral composition: men are humorally hot and dry, while women are humorally cold and moist. These are the basic assumptions from which recommendations for food and drink are derived.

Given that the *Trotula* specifically addressed women's health, it makes sense that most of the recommendations are concerned with gynaecological and obstetric conditions. Much of medieval medicine was concerned with conditions experienced by both men and women: fevers, poor digestion, infections, disease, headaches, and other common medical complaints. Treatments could be adjusted according to the humoral balance of the patient, but by and large the treatment strategy didn't change significantly whether the patient was male or female. To talk primarily about women's health, therefore, meant addressing the female reproductive system: menses, pregnancy, birth, lactation, infertility, uterine complaints, and so forth. *On the Conditions of Women* covers multiple gynaecological concerns: menstrual disturbances, pathologies of the womb, itching of the vagina, infertility and conception, signs of pregnancy, dietary regimens for pregnant women, and difficulties in birth or the post-partum period (Green 2002).

The menses in women are explained in the context of Greco-Roman medicine. Menstrual flow results from an excess in 'bad and superfluous humours'. These humours are the result of incomplete concoction due to women's cold and moist nature. The Greeks, and later writers in the history of humoral theory, saw the menses as a purgative, and beneficial to women. Thus, an excess of menstrual flow, as well as its paucity or absence, were of concern to medical writers, the author of the *Book on the Conditions of Women* certainly among them. In fact, aberrations in normal menstrual flow were thought to cause a variety of symptoms and illnesses, including a loss of appetite for food and drink, vomiting, or pica – all of these involving digestive disturbances (Green 2002, 66). Other digestive symptoms could be diarrhoea, dysentery, or dropsy. Sometimes improper menstrual flow could also be caused, in part, by diet: rich foods in excess could cause thickening or coagulation of the humours, which might themselves impede menstrual flow. Paucity might also be addressed with food and drink, with pungent foods such as onions, leeks, pepper, garlic, and cumin, consumed with strong wine (Green 2002, 69).

Excessive menstrual flow was attributed to a number of things, mostly related to an overabundance of blood in the system, and especially in the uterus. One possible cause was overindulgence in food and drink, which could create blood in excess. Threats to fertility caused by a corpulent body would become increasingly recognized into the Early Modern period

(Toulalan 2014), and were already recognized to a certain extent in the Middle Ages. Excessive menstrual flow was also attributed to blood heated to excess by an overabundance of bile, or the admixture of salty phlegm. It could sometimes be caused by a defect of heat that impedes digestion of fluids, thus making them flow into the blood in excess, according to the Greco-Roman tradition. While bleeding was prescribed as a possible remedy (as it was for many illnesses to which humoral causes could be attributed), or medicines could be prescribed, changes in diet could also be effective in ameliorating the humoral condition leading to the increase in blood volume during menses. *On the Conditions of Women* suggests chicken, fresh fish, barley bread, and barley water to lessen menstrual flow (Green 2002, 70).

Greek theories about diet used to address humoral abnormalities are evident here. The recommendation for the consumption of chicken, fish and barley – considered easily digested foods – likely comes from the idea that women were unable to concoct (digest, but here with the literal meaning of cooking) their food as well as men, because of their lower humoral heat (Green 2002, 20). We have seen this recommendation in previously mentioned texts. For Greek medical writers, the only way for women to purge themselves of excessive waste, which they retained due to their cold nature and inability to fully concoct their food, was through the menses. When the menses were excessive, the recommendation for easily digested food would, theoretically, reduce the amount of waste needing to be eliminated (Green 2002, 19). There are also recommendations for prescribing 'cold' and styptic foods to treat 'descent of the womb', based on the Greek idea that the womb could become detached from its original position, wandering through the body and causing distressing symptoms. Its opposite complaint was called 'suffocation of the womb', when the uterus was said to move upward, making it difficult to breathe. Stemming largely from Hippocratic gynaecology, writings in the Hippocratic tradition offer numerous remedies for moving the womb back into place. Most are not dietary, but cold and styptic foods would theoretically reduce blood flow and therefore be more likely to keep the womb in place (Faraone 2011).

The recommendation for a certain diet for pregnant women was also present in Greek and Arabic medicine. For example, around 900 CE, 'Rhazes was one of the first Arabic writers to include a pregnancy-regimen in his regimen-cycle of the *Liber de medicina ad Al-mansorem*' (Weiss-Amer 1993, 13). Dietary recommendations were also no doubt present in the practical oral tradition of midwives and other women healers. Light and digestible foods make sense in terms of a humoral understanding of the body, but also practically, because pregnant women often experience nausea and heartburn.

The *Trotula* also recommends consuming light and easily digestible foods during labour. Although in contemporary hospital settings in the United States, women are often kept from eating any solid food during labour, other cultures have traditional foods which should be eaten during labour and after birth. One recommendation (Green 2002, 65) suggests light and digestible foods – egg yolks, poultry and fish – as protection against a difficult birth. The general idea here seems to be that women in a delicate condition should eat what was considered appropriate for invalids, as we have already seen.[2] It should also be noted that the advice in the *Book of the Conditions of Women* was intended for more professionally trained doctors in the literate tradition, whose clients were wealthy enough to consult a physician. Poultry and fish had long been recommended as appropriate food for the constitution of the aristocracy (Henisch 1990 [1976]).

Recommendations for producing an appropriately abundant milk supply of good nutritional value and of the right consistency is found in 'On Choosing a Wet Nurse' (Green 2002, 85). Nursing women are advised against eating foods 'hot' in nature, as well as foods that would impede the flow of milk – i.e. styptic foods. As theoretical medicine taught that milk was made directly from blood (Åström 2015), styptic substances meant to impede blood flow were contraindicated. Sweet, bland, and starchy foods are recommended for thickening milk and increasing milk production[3], while physical labor and wine are recommended to thin milk.

From *On Treatments for Women*

The second book of the *Trotula, On Treatments for Women,* is most likely to have been recorded by Trota or her students. There is less of the theoretical medicine found in *Conditions of Women* (although it is certainly not absent), and more practical remedies, such as might be written by a practicing physician whose training might have been partially theoretical, but was informed by observation and practice. There is less theoretical background

2 See Bald's Leechbook III: 'A pregnant woman is to be earnestly warned that she should eat nothing salty or sweet, nor drink beer, nor eat swine's flesh nor anything fat, nor drink to intoxication …' (Wallis, 2010, 125)

3 This recommendation relies on ideas akin to sympathetic magic, or like produces like. Here, thick, sweet food should be consumed in order to stimulate the production of thick, sweet milk.

for each recommendation, and more emphasis on practical treatment. The recommendations are not arranged in any particular order, looking more like a notebook or record an individual physician might create over time.

The topics covered are similar to those found in *Conditions of Women*, but are more wide-ranging (Green 2002). For example, aside from the normal complaints about menstrual disorders, pregnancy, infertility, and the like, there are also treatments that really seem to have nothing much to do with women in particular, including difficulty in urination, treatment for 'stone' – possibly kidney or bladder stones – sunburn, dental issues, lesions, eye pain, deafness and worm of the ears, and haemorrhoids. Other remedies directed at women alone have to do with constriction of the vagina so that a woman could appear to be a virgin, removing freckles, whitening the face, and removing wrinkles.

Dietary recommendations are relatively scarce, involving only three non-specific recommendations for good wine and wholesome food. More reflective of practice-based, practical Salernitan medical tradition, there are two recommendations for helping fat women, both phlegmatic and dropsical, to conceive. Both actually list a regimen of baths, sweats, and other treatments to induce weight loss, but still recommend nourishing food.

Hildegard of Bingen

Hildegard was born in the Rhineland in 1098 and died in 1179, her life spanning the 'Twelfth Century Renaissance' (Sweet 1999). She was the tenth child of well-to-do parents, and was promised to the religious life by her parents early on, as a 'tithe' to the Church. She entered the monastery at Disibodenberg at age fourteen. Unusually, this monastery was for both men and women, each living in a different part of the monastery. This may have given her greater access to a wide variety of texts than she might otherwise have had in a strictly female monastery. At the age of 38, she was elected as the *magistra* or abbess. Hildegard began her writing after this point, beginning with the book *Scivias*, in which she explained some of her visions. At the age of 50, she opted to leave to start her own monastery about twenty miles away, in the Rupertsburg area of Bingen, where she was extremely successful at attracting entrants. She was best known for her visions, and also gained some reputation as a healer. She would remain abbess of Rupertsburg for thirty years, writing on a wide variety of subjects and earning a reputation as an important mystic. She was visited by noted religious and secular figures, leaving the monastery from time to time to preach (Sweet 1999; Cadden 1984).

Hildegard on natural philosophy and medicine

Hildegard's two works on natural philosophy and medicine, known today as *Physica* and *Causae et curae*, grew from both her wide-ranging intellectual curiosity and her probable experience as a healer. They were written between CE 1151 and 1158, after she had begun to receive recognition from such important church figures as Bernard of Clairvaux and Pope Eugenius III (Bingen 2006). This point is somewhat in doubt: while some authors, like Rachel Sweet, enthusiastically endorse the notion that Hildegard was a gifted healer experienced in both Galenic medicine and traditional herbal lore (herself an avid gardener particularly astute in the cultivation of medicinal herbs), others do not find sufficient evidence for this assertion. Some scholars feel there is not sufficient evidence to definitively assign authorship to these works, most notably Laurence Moulinier (Stuard 2007), or that her own relatively aristocratic status prevented her from heavy duties in the garden (Rawcliffe 2008). It is likely true, however, that she became locally well-known for her healing ability and was visited for exorcism and healing as well as for her counsel (Bingen 2006, ii). She was beatified by the Church in 1326, becoming a doctor of the Church, but was only canonized in 2012 under Pope Benedict, himself a German.

Physica and *Causae et curae* are not treatises on medicine or natural philosophy exclusively; instead Hildegard places her interpretations of the human body, its functioning and illness, within the much broader cosmology of her overall, somewhat idiosyncratic theology, though that is not the primary focus of these two works (Bingen 2006). In fact, some of this idiosyncrasy can be found in her understanding of the humours:

> 'Humours' and their balance are central to Hildegard's theories, but her discussion of the humours has greater affinity with Eastern medicine than with the traditional Greek humoral pathology. To the Greeks, hot is choler, or yellow bile; dry is blood; moist is phlegm; and cold is black bile. Hildegard distinguishes between the dry, damp, foamy, and cool humours. Any humour exceeding its measure endangers a person (Throop 2006, 5).

While she is in accord with Hippocratic medicine in the number of four humours, Hildegard writes that the two preeminent humours are derived from phlegm, and the other two from *livores*, or dark humours resembling slime (Throop 2006, 5). Hildegard also attributes human illness to the fall of Adam and the expulsion from Paradise, as Adam and Eve were created by God in perfect health. This is an interpretation consistent with ecclesiastical tradition.

While mentioning some conditions and diseases specific to women, Hildegard does not focus on women's medicine *per se*, but rather on her understanding of the human body, its place within creation, and how humoral makeup can affect health and illness. Her understanding of the differences between the sexes do not strictly follow either Galen or Aristotelian models (Cadden 1984, 173).

Dietary recommendations from *Causae et Curae*

In discussing how sexual relations should be approached moderately (unlike how the glutton approaches food), and at the right time, Hildegard cautions as well against actual gluttony, saying gluttony and intoxication can lead to twisted limbs and leprosy (Bingen 2006, pp. 15-16).

This recommendation for moderation is present in more standard medical texts, but in Hildegard's case is also informed by Church teachings internalized throughout her monastic life. The Church taught that gluttony was sinful, demonstrating a lack of self-mastery, and Hildegard echoes this teaching in her medical commentary (Bingen 2006, 31). The Church's stance on sex also reinforced the idea that a Christian works at all times for self-mastery of bodily appetites. Virginity was the preferred state; sexual relations ideally should only take place within marriage for procreative purposes rather than simple pleasure.

In reference to conception, Hildegard maintained that a person's humoral composition would affect his or her ability to procreate. In addition, the phase of the moon, the position of the sun in the zodiac, and even the weather conditions could also play a role in conception. Each individual's humoral composition also dictated how much, and how strongly, food and drink would affect his or her health. The conditions of conception would help determine the health and predilections of the resulting offspring. Those with the best health and temperament are conceived during the full moon when the weather is neither too hot nor too cold (Bingen 2006, 80).

Other sections of *Causae* address how a person conceived when the sun is in Cancer cannot easily digest raw fruits and vegetables; for this person, food should be cooked or tempered by a condiment, like salt or vinegar, making the food more digestible[4]. She cautioned against overindulging in

4 Tying information about the zodiac to health and constitution was itself an old and common practice. The zodiac was not viewed as it is now, but rather as a key to understanding God's creation through links between the heavens and people's lives (Retief and Cilliers 2010).

'raw, uncooked or half cooked food' or food that is 'excessively fatty, heavy, dry, or desiccated', as these foods are all difficult to digest and tend to result in harmful *livor* in the body.

In discussing the causes of gout, Hildegard draws upon ancient Greek ideas about menstruation and the elimination of waste, or excess humours. She notes that gout is caused by eating 'various, luxurious foods', especially by someone with soft, delicate flesh. Men who overindulge in harmful food – without balancing it by eating a greater quantity of healthy food – suffer from gout. The excess humour descends to the lower part of the body, turns to *livor,* and causes pain and difficulty in walking. For women, however, their unique bodily functions could mitigate the harmful effects, as menstruation would help to eliminate some of the harmful humours. This echoes, at least in part, ideas discussed earlier that go all the way back to ancient Greece. Obesity during pregnancy, however, when there was no menstruation to purge the body of bad humours, could result in difficult and unproductive labour (Bingen 2006, 89). This is why, according to *Causae,* women should not overindulge in rich, luxurious foods.

Hildegard undertakes a descriptive and explanatory approach to the processes of the human body and of the effect of the 'non-naturals' upon the body. Since this work is not specifically a gynaecological text, nor is it solely a book of remedies, Hildegard presents her own interpretation of natural philosophy – drawn to some extent from knowledge of, and probably access to, medical and philosophical texts – combined with her own theologically-inflected interpretation. She explains the importance of food and drink to the proper functioning of the body, whether male or female.

Hildegard wrote general advice on eating and drinking in the maintenance of health. She rarely gave different guidelines for men and women, but they do occasionally arise in her work. She also had a tendency to talk about cold, warm, and hot foods not only in terms of their humoral composition, but also in terms of the temperature at which they are consumed. A fasting person, for example, should eat grains and flour, which are humorally dry. However, Hildegard also advises that the first food consumed after a fast should be eaten at a warm temperature, so the stomach is heated (aiding digestion/concoction). Cold food, she cautions, cools the stomach so that it impedes digestion, and prevents warming from thermally warm foods if the cold is eaten first. However, she also cautions against the consumption of fruit and other moist foods first, as these are humorally cold, rather than necessarily cold in temperature (Bingen 2006, 95).

She also makes a distinction between the dietary habits for a healthy person versus someone who is ill. For example, Hildegard recommends that a healthy person not consume the morning meal until just before midday in order to promote good digestion. However, for someone who is sick or weak, their own strength is not sufficient to last until midday, so they should eat earlier. At night, she advises all people who take a second meal to consume it early enough to allow time for a walk before retiring for the evening (Bingen 2006, 95).

Hildegard does make one distinction between men and women in dietary recommendations: 'A woman has many more noxious humours and more noxious lymph in her body than a man' (Bingen 2006, 99). As was commonly believed in the written medical tradition, menstrual periods would help eliminate some of these noxious substances. Blood-letting, a common method of addressing humoral imbalance in the Middle Ages, was also recommended (Bingen 2006, 99).

The idea that a proper diet consisted of moderation in food and drink, and alternating physically hot and cold as well as humorally hot and cold substances is present throughout her dietary recommendations. Some of them also reference Hildegard's particular take on Greek medicine, overlaid with her experience as a woman religious. We can see the influence of living a monastic life in her stance on excessive food and drink, which leads to 'delectation', a euphemism for sexual desire. In the *Trotula*, the concern is more related to fertility and difficulty in childbirth. Excessive food and drink, like excessive happiness or emotion, creates a 'stormy fervour' in the blood, which travels to the genital organs. While Hildegard seems to condone sexual intercourse under the proper conditions for the promotion of a healthy baby, she frowns on delectation for its own sake, warning that this excessive heat can lead to unnatural desires, particularly on the part of men[5]. For the semen to be strong, Hildegard writes, it must be warmed not just by the man, but by the presence of a woman as well – otherwise it would be thin and watery. This seems to be a teaching against masturbation, though not mentioned explicitly (Bingen 2006, 111-112).

These recommendations are consistent with Church teachings on the relationship between gluttony and sexual incontinence. While the *Trotula* and *Causae* are both related to the legacy of Greek medicine, the influence of religious teachings, a preference for Aristotle's thesis that women do not need to have sex to maintain health, access to more limited or general texts, efforts at theological consistence, and individual interpretation are evident in Hildegard's work, but absent from the *Trotula*.

5 Within the text, Hildegard sometimes seems to refer to homosexual sex, and at other times intercourse with animals. Both were considered sinful.

Physica

There is some overlap between *Causae et curae* and *Physica*, though they have different purposes. The authorship of *Physica* is not disputed. It is essentially a book of characteristics for all of creation, broken down into categories and evaluated for their usefulness and potential to affect human health and the humours, as Hildegard understood them. In *Physica*, she also notes which things are useful as remedies and gives some idea of how to use them, although the recipes included in the work are not always very specific. As always, she aims for a balance of the humours, and moderation in all things (Bingen 1998, 5-6).

As with *Causae et cure,* Hildegard's dietary recommendations tend to the general, rather than being specifically gender-based, although she does mention ailments specific to either women or men in some of her suggested remedies. The nine books of the *Physica* are divided into plants, elements, trees, stone, fish, birds, animals, reptiles, and metals. Listings within each category are not exhaustive, but they do cover a wide variety of items. Her writing once again reflects her own idiosyncratic understanding of the world and the usefulness of all things in God's creation.

Let us take one example from the section on plants, the entry on galingale[6]. Galingale (*Alpinia officinarum*) is a member of the ginger family, and its rhizome was one of the primary spices used in medieval European cooking. Although indigenous to southeast Asia, it would have been available to anyone with access to a spice market. Hildegard describes galingale as completely hot, with no humoral coldness. Accordingly, it could be used in spring water to counteract a high fever, or boiled in wine for bad humours, heart pain, or a weak heart. It can also be used in conjunction with fennel, nutmeg, and feverfew in the treatment of stinking breath. There follows a list of remedies, seemingly unrelated to the use of galingale (Bingen 1998, 15-16).

The entry for galingale, though one of the longer ones, is typical of Hildegard's writing in *Physica*. She ascribes a humoral nature to all things, noting whether or not they have medicinal value. She is very clear on what makes substances healthful or medicinal, also pointing out items with no medicinal use or that are harmful when used or ingested. For example, in her entry for the mascel tree, she notes it is harmful in all cases (Bingen 1998, 128).

6 'Galingal' is another common spelling.

Alcohol consumption

Let us consider another consumable item, alcohol. When not taken in excess, alcohol was considered a healthful drink for most people, and in fact was exceedingly common as a standard beverage. It was part of an overall diet promoting good health. Wine seems to have been especially valued, but one sees recommendations for different kinds of wine (red, white, sweet, strong, gentle, old, young), as well as for ale, beer, mead, claret, and hydromel in a variety of medical texts and regimens. The type of alcohol recommended typically depends on region and socio-economic status. Alcohol, especially wine, was considered a warming substance, but also a tempering one – its heat was not thought too harsh (at least when diluted with water), and could temper both hot and cold substances to make them more manageable for the body. The *Trotula* recommends wine almost exclusively as a fermented beverage, but if we consult a sixteenth century guide to women's health (BL Sloane 2463), partially based on the *Trotula*, we note that ale and beer appear far more frequently than they did in the original. This difference is owing to consumption habits in sixteenth century England, where wine was a luxury item and beer and ale were far more commonly consumed (Rowland 1981).

Alcohol was often used as a solvent for herbs or other substances; herbs could be both heated and processed in alcohol, or a substance could simply be added to alcohol for consumption. Many recipes call for herbs processed in wine, usually cooked, although sometimes further processing occurs. While assessing herbal medicine is not the aim of this chapter, an illustrative example might prove useful. In 'On Retention of the Menses' in *Book on the Conditions of Women*, the author advises:

> All diuretic substances are good for her, such as fennel, spikenard, wild celery, cumin, cowbane, caraway, parsley, and similar things. All these herbs together or individually are useful when cooked in wine or drunk with honey (Green 2002, 67).

This direction is given repeatedly throughout all three books of the *Trotula*, and seems to have been a very common way to extract the active substances from herbs. This is not the only method of processing herbs for medicine, but is one of the most frequent. Wine itself would have been the most common drink available in Salerno, besides water, and given what we know about diet in the region, would have been consumed in various grades and dilutions, but nearly always when eating. This is in contrast to more northern areas, where ale or beer were more commonly consumed. Hildegard lived in what is now Germany, where beer and ale were readily available as a common drink; Salerno, in southern Italy, was an exclusively wine-drinking area.

Three female conditions for which alcohol is mentioned as a specific remedy are lactation (prescribed when the milk was too 'thick'), excessive menstrual bleeding (wine and beer strengthen the woman, making her better able to retain her blood), and lack of menstrual bleeding (the consumption of light food and wine will render the blood less constricted).

Problems of milk production could be serious: failure to produce milk, or to produce adequate milk, could be deadly to an infant unless the parents were wealthy enough to afford a wet-nurse (usually reserved for aristocratic families). Increasingly through the Middle Ages, the kind of milk a woman produced was also thought to be related to her character: women of a bad or sinful nature produced inferior quality milk. According to *De secretis mulierum*, the quality of a woman's milk could also be based on whether she was carrying a boy or a girl. Carrying a girl caused inferior quality milk (Laurent 1989, 123). The *Trotula,* however, based its recommendation for milk production strictly on the basis of physiological conditions, rather than making moral judgements about the quality of a woman's milk. It recommends delicate food and exercise, light wine, and vinegar to resolve the problem of milk that was 'too thick' (Green 2002, 85). Hildegard makes similar dietary recommendations.

Regarding paucity of the menses, strong wine should be given in order to increase the menstrual flow. 'Let her drink strong wine if she has no pain in the head nor any nervous disorder nor any fever, because wine is harmful in any fever'. Strong wine would warm the body and digestive system, thus perhaps loosening coagulated substances or improving humoral heat so that food could be more completely concocted (Green 2002, 69). The treatises are in agreement that excessive or improper blood flow sometimes requires humorally cold substances, or substances that strengthen the body enough to retain the excessive blood flow.

Just as food and wine could play a role in helping to lessen excessive blood flow – either by providing proper nourishment to strengthen the woman, or as a vehicle for processing or giving medicines – so wine could also be used to prompt absent or blocked menses. In the writings under discussion, the provocation of menstruation for the purpose of aborting a foetus is never mentioned (though perhaps it could not have been safely mentioned due to Church teachings). Absent or delayed menses are considered a problem if they prevent the elimination of waste material, are caused by or are symptomatic of infertility, or cause discomfort to the woman.

Alcohol could also be used topically, usually with some other substance within it, to heal from the exterior in. It is used as a softener for body parts that have become hard due to illness or engorgement, and is recommended by both Trota and Hildegard for a softening of a prolapsed uterus before reinsertion.

One further use for wine was as part of a fumigation, a common treatment for problems associated with the female reproductive organs. For a fumigation, substances were heated until they produced fragrance, smoke, or steam. The woman would then stand or sit over the substances to allow the beneficial vapours to enter her vagina and, presumably, her womb. A prolapsed or 'wandering' womb might also be sent back to its proper place with a fumigation of foul-smelling substances from which the uterus would naturally recoil (Green 2002, 97). Alcohol might also be used in the preparation of herbs for a poultice, or to make a medical bath.

Hildegard on alcohol

Hildegard emphasizes numerous times that drink is as vital as food to the functioning of the body, as moisture is necessary for the proper balance of humours. Thirst, she says, must be satisfied and drink taken with food, otherwise a person would become 'heavy in mind and body' (2006, 93). When a person is dehydrated, the food in the body dries and rots. She cautions, however, that the proper time to drink is not immediately upon waking, especially if one is subject to gout. Drinking while still sleepy would 'bring on infirmities, and stir up his blood and humours in excessive storms' (2006, 91). As soon as one is completely awake, one should drink according to thirst. In this case, the drink should be wine or beer, as water would at this point be detrimental to the blood and humours (Bingen 2006, 94). Wine or beer is recommended for those who tend to be immoderate in behaviour, and wine should be drunk on an empty stomach. If wine is not available, then beer made from barley or rye is advised. If neither is available, then bread and water should be cooked together and strained, and drunk lukewarm.

Despite Hildegard's enthusiasm for wine, she cautions against drinking expensive or strong wine, as they are detrimental to the blood and veins, acting more as a purgative than a drink. Wine, she noted, can also cause excessive urination. Expensive wine should be moderated by placing bread in it or diluting it with water. Hildegard does mention that Heunisch wine is not strong enough to be harmful, and does not need these precautions. The Heunisch varietal was considered a lesser grape, and was used to make wine especially in Germanic regions[7].

Further cautions against overindulgence in wine are found in *Causae et curae*. 'Wine is the blood of the earth', says Hildegard (2006, 115). She says that drinking wine that is too strong can 'scorch' a person, with particularly ill effect upon the bladder. Essentially, wine should always be drunk diluted with water; even a relatively gentle wine, like Heunisch wine, is more beneficial when cut with water. A person who is ill should not drink wine unless it is mixed with water. Hildegard seems to have considered beer to be gentler than wine, so it was not necessary to dilute it. Again, drinking an excess of wine in particular (along with overeating) had a tendency to stir up lust. Even the rules of Lenten abstinence were derived from the idea that Lenten foods, such as fish, vegetables, and bread, were less likely to lead to lust than strong wine, red meat, and luxurious or fatty foods (Vigarello 2010). Drinking to excess, according to Hildegard, made the blood dissipate and run wildly in the body, causing an untamed intellect, mistaken perceptions, and the submersion of rationality (2006, 122). Should a woman who was nursing, be it as a wet-nurse or a mother, consume strong wine, the milk would turn fetid and cause bladder stones in the infant (Bingen 2006, 129-30). Still, Hildegard thought wine could have a beneficial effect, as it 'heals and cheers a person with its good heat and great power" (2006, 122).

Beer, commonly consumed in Germany, was also beneficial, and perhaps gentler than wine. 'Beer thickens a person's flesh, and gives his face a beautiful colour, because of the strength and beneficial juice of its grain' (Bingen 2006, 122). Hildegard considered it a healthier drink than water, which could weaken the body and cause *livor* or slime around the lungs. Water was fine as an occasional drink for healthy people, but was not generally recommended. In addition, while Hildegard believed leprosy could be caused by consuming meat, spoiled milk, and strong wine, it could be avoided by drinking beer and eating bread and vegetables (perhaps not incidentally the standard monastic diet) (2006, 130).

7 The Heunisch grape variety, Weißer Heunisch, is also known as Gouais blanc. It is a rare grape variety today, but was commonly grown in Germany during the Middle Ages. It was considered milder than Frankish grape varieties, also available at the time (Wein-Plus 2018).

Similarities and contrasts in the *Trotula* and the works of Hildegard

Causae at curae and *Physica*, aside from containing general recommendations on diet to promote health (which sometimes includes exhortations to refrain from overindulgence), use food as a treatment for specific diseases and conditions. As in the *Trotula*, and indeed much of the written medical tradition, sometimes the food itself is the medicine, and a humorally adjusted diet might allow the humours of the body to return to their proper balance. Also as in the *Trotula,* herbs are sometimes eaten as they are or are made into a juice, but are often processed using wine and heat to render them more effective. Medicine itself could be processed with alcohol, and food could be used as an adjunct to medication, provided the proper food was combined with the proper medication.

This recommendation is typical of Hildegard's medicine. *Physica* also mirrors to some extent the variety of plants, medicine, and diet promoted for health in the *Trotula*. Not all the recipes are the same, of course, but there is enough similarity to speculate that Hildegard and the author(s) of the *Trotula* probably had access to some medical manuscripts derived from the same Greco-Roman tradition. Victoria Sweet argues that Hildegard was an expert on herbs herself, and spent time in the priory garden, and using herbs to treat people who came to the abbey seeking medical help (2006). While Sweet's analysis has been criticized for overstating the likelihood that Hildegard was herself an avid gardener and spent a great deal of time treating illness, it is certainly possible that her knowledge of healing herbs stretched beyond what she was taught informally or read in herbals.

If we examine some of Hildegard's treatments specific to women's complaints we find treatments similar, although not identical, to those in the *Trotula*. For example, 'obstruction of the menses' is addressed several times in *Causae et curae*, including a long section outlining proper treatments. Specific instructions are given for the making of a sauna bath in which an afflicted woman should sit on a particular combination of herbs, and place them again around her navel. Hildegard counsels that the herbs are most effective when warmed, and have the effect of softening the reproductive organs and opening the veins. She takes care to call for the use of river water from an outdoor area that receives both sun and wind, as she thought this water more healthful due to its proximity to the elements. Hot tiles are used to warm the bath because the tiles themselves are formed in the heat of a kiln or firing, and thus have healthful warming properties, according to Hildegard. The second part of the treatment for obstruction of the menses involves crushing a number of herbs and spices and cooking them in wine, then adding honey to good wine to make a claret. Hildegard believed that all herbs, spices, and wines have warming properties, and this heat would in turn encourage the menstrual blood to flow. Along with these two treatments are a recommendation for mush or porridge made from eggs, lard, and lovage juice the woman should eat before and after meals. The food the patient consumes should be sweet, and she should drink wine or water that has been boiled and cooled, and avoid beef and other 'coarse' foods (Bingen 2006, 149-150).

Compare Hildegard's advice to the prescription found in the *Treatments for Women* treatise in the *Trotula*, where the recommendation is to pulverize the roots of a red willow and mix them with wine or water and cook. The potion should be served lukewarm after the woman wakes in the morning. The *Trotula* also recommends consuming small wafers made of madder, marsh mallow, barley flour, and egg white (Green 2002, 90).

Hildegard places emphasis on where the best water is found, and why certain types of water are more healthful than others. She is also more explicit about the humoral reasoning behind her prescribed treatment. Both authors recommend making drinks from plants cooked in water or wine. They both recommend food that is gentle for the stomach. While Hildegard mentions an herbal bath and hot herbs, the *Trotula* calls for a fumigation; both recommendations indicate that heat increases the beneficial effects of the herbs, and that smoke or steam should be allowed to enter the womb. This indicates similar philosophies about the proper processing of herbs and ways of moving them into the body through ingestion, fumigation, or vapours. The *Trotula* recommendation appears in the section most likely to be from a practicing physician, and the absence of humoral explanation for the treatment is more in line with its emphasis on empirical treatments, rather than theoretical ones. If we look at *Conditions of Women*, the first book of the *Trotula*, the author often gives more information on the reasoning behind the treatments.

In *Conditions of Women*, the sections dealing with retention of menses are considerably longer, and make reference to Galen and theoretical medicine. The treatments include blood-letting, remedies for constipation including herbal baths, processing herbs with honey or cooked in wine, fumigation, the application of medicinal herbs pounded to a paste directly to the abdomen, being given medicinal drinks in the bath, the making of vaginal suppositories from carded wool dipped in natron or bull gall and juice of wild celery or hyssop, and the insertion of a pessary containing medicine (2002, 67-68).

There is some overlap in the herbs recommended in the *Trotula* and *Causae* for the obstruction or retention of the menses, but the overlap is not extensive. Hildegard mentions the use of anise, feverfew, mullein, bearberry, yarrow, rue, birthwort, lovage, dittany, *apertum* clove, and white pepper (Bingen 2006, 149-150). In *Conditions of Women*, the herbs mentioned include: calamint, catmint, mint, myrtle berry, fleawort, birthwort, laurel berry, fennel, spikenard, wild celery, cumin, cowbane, caraway, parsley, mugwort, deadly carrot, sermountain, sage, oregano, savin, balm, pennyroyal, dill, anise, summer savoury, lovage, chickweed, yellow flag, hemlock, castoreum, sea wormwood, and hyssop. (Green 2002, 67-68) The selection from *Treatments for Women* mentions only red willow, madder, and marsh mallow (Green 2002, 90). Of these recommendations, there is no overlap between Hildegard and the author of *Treatments for Women* and only anise and birthwort between *Conditions of Women* and Hildegard. Why might this be?

First, while Hildegard probably had access to some medical texts, we do not know what they were, although they probably had some relationship to the tradition of Greco-Roman medicine. The *Alphabet of Galen,* derived from the written tradition of herblore well before Hildegard lived, has this to say about anise:

> The best anise is Cretan, then Egyptian ... Anise is used for its excellent softening, warming, and diuretic properties. Its seed is similar to hemlock. When drunk it stimulates and increases lactation for infants, and its fragrance is sweet (Everett 2014, p. 157).

This manuscript, really a compilation of a number of different Latin manuscripts from the seventh to the eleventh centuries, contains pharmacological knowledge most likely based upon the Greek tradition. This is the lineage of the *Trotula*. The description of the pharmacological uses of anise are consistent with the goal of softening and warming the uterus, thus encouraging the flow of the menses. Regarding birthwort[8], the *Alphabet of Galen* says:

> Birthwort can be either spherical or long, but the spherical type is better for medical uses, and this type should not be used when it is old, pungent, dry, slightly thickened, or has a bitter taste. It is added to plasters and used to fill and seal hollow wounds. It is an antidote for bites and some types of internal poisoning (Everett 2014, 159).

8 *Aristolochia sp.*

While the specific use for retention of the menses is not mentioned in the *Alphabet*, its name probably comes from the doctrine of signatures, since it resembles the shape of a human uterus. The name birthwort itself is derived from the Greek for 'best birth' (*Aristolochia*), so we can infer its use to stimulate labour or treat blockages after labour were well known.

The fact that there is only a two ingredient overlap between Hildegard and the *Conditions of Women* may also suggest that Hildegard's herbal recommendations are a result, not just of some knowledge of Greek pharmacology, but perhaps much greater knowledge either of local or regional herb-lore, or her own unique interpretation of the uses for various herbs. This may be evidence for the use of folk medicine in some of Hildegard's suggested treatments, as they do suggest local knowledge.

It is somewhat frustrating (though consistent with the literary tradition) that so much of the advice on diet, both food and drink, in the *Trotula* lack a specific theoretical explanation. We are left to guess the specific humoral action of each recommendation, and it is possible that many of these recommendations arise out of simple tradition in the medical texts, which had either become divorced from the theoretical tradition, or had never been part of it in the first place. It is also possible that some were influenced by folk tradition. In other words, there is humoral theory on the one hand, and a collection of specific recipes and treatments on the other, and the two are not always directly related to or consistent with each other in the *Trotula*.

The medical school at Salerno would, by the fourteenth century, be eclipsed by other, larger, university-based medical schools. Medicine, now taught at many universities, became increasingly professionalized. (Wallis, 2010, xxiii) However, the *Trotula* continued to be a popular work, found in translation in other parts of Europe, through the fifteenth century. As a relatively early site of Arabic influence on Western medical theory, through the systemization of Greek ideas in Arabic writing translated into Latin, we can see the influences of Greek and Arabic medical understanding overlaid on the indigenous traditions of the southern Italian peninsula.

It is also significant that the text was, correctly or incorrectly, attributed to a female author, and was respected even after professional medicine became almost exclusively male- dominated. Were women in medicine thought to be most appropriately concerned with the health of other women? That was certainly true in the tradition of midwives and wise women, most closely identified with folk medicine, or medicine not part of the written tradition.

Were Hildegard and Trota practitioners of folk medicine?

Hildegard wrote to record her healing knowledge, but also as a way to systematize her theology and apply it to God's creation, to show the microcosm of the body as situated within and allied with the macrocosm of the universe. The Greek writers certainly had no such aim and theoretical medicine as it developed in Europe was only loosely associated with Christian theology. Religion does make its way into later medieval texts that cover medicine or natural philosophy, and changes in religious beliefs and emphases can certainly be found within them. For example, attitudes towards women on the part of ecclesiastical writers are blindingly evident as early writing on women's health in the *Trotula* ends up two centuries later in the anti-feminist work *De secretis mulierum* (Lemay 1992; Green 2000b).

The works of the *Trotula* also originate in the area of Salerno, site of Europe's first medical school and renowned in its day for advancements in medicine. The site of the intersection of Latinate medicine and influence from Arab and Jewish medical writers, the reputation and geographical position of Salerno and the rise of the professionalization of medicine helped ensure that the ideas in the *Trotula* would spread and continue, especially set within the context of the development of medieval medicine. Hildegard, with her location in the Rhineland in the cities of Disibodenberg and Rupertsburg, was in a relative backwater. Her medical works, while connected to theoretical Greco-Roman medicine, did not have a strong or lasting effect on European academic medicine. While her reputation as a theologian and musical composer survived, interest in her medicine was shorter lived, at least until its revival in the twentieth century as a kind of guide to alternative and natural health in Germany (Micke and Hübner 2009).

Why then should we consider the work of Hildegard when looking at dietary recommendations in European medicine, primarily derived from Greek roots? First, because Hildegard does stand out as the likely author of two medical works. Works of medicine written by women are exceedingly rare in this period, in contrast to books of remedies collected and written by largely aristocratic women that come many centuries later (Fissell 2008), and Hildegard's works should not go entirely ignored. Here is a woman who had the confidence (and later the support of the Church) to write on a variety of subjects, including a wide-ranging theory of medicine. Her inventive mind saw order in God's universe. Second, there is evidence that Hildegard was, in fact, sought out for her healing ability, no doubt due to her knowledge, but also to the religious component of her ability to heal, an area in which holy women were equal to or greater than men (Ritchey 2014). She is interesting in her own right, and in the broader picture of women who do 'bodywork', or care for the human body in myriad ways.

There is also the possibility that Hildegard's medical works contain, in addition to her own idiosyncratic take on medicine and healing, elements of regional folk medicine. While medicine derived from the Hippocratic Corpus was generally hostile to folk medicine or traditional remedies, other strands of medicine were not (Riddle 2013). When I compared treatments for the retention of the menses between *Causae et curae*, *Conditions of Women*, and *Treatments for Women*, it is clear that Hildegard's herblore was divergent from that in the *Trotula*. Whether or not the case for Hildegard as a master of herb-lore is overstated, there is something to the idea that she came by her knowledge of herbs in some hands-on way. As she does not rely heavily on the written medical tradition, it is possible she drew from regional folk medicine and traditional knowledge.

How can we demonstrate such a thing? If we compare Hildegard's treatment of herbs to those found in the *Alphabet of Galen* we see significant variances compared to the content of the *Trotula*. For example, Hildegard prescribes sage, bryony, and rue for intestinal pain because of their humoral heat and warming properties. The *Alphabet of Galen*, by contrast, states that sage is astringent, bryony is sharp and warming and should be used in salves, and that rue is useful for coughs, neck pain, stimulates urine and menstruation, and can be used as an abortifacient, in addition to being useful for fortifying the stomach (Everett 2014, 225, 177, 319). If we look in *Physica* for these three substances, we find that sage is hot and dry, and works against noxious humours (1998, 36), that bryony is hot and useless for humans except in the case of poisoning (1998, 28), and that rue has temperate heat and moisture, checks 'excessive passion' (i.e. lust), and helps dissipate noxious humours (1998, 37-38). It is possible that Hildegard did not have access to this standard book of herblore. The differences in use could be due to her own idiosyncratic interpretation, but may be equally due to regional variation in herbal medicine and the traditional medicine of her region.

Early Greek medicine itself was at least partially based on the traditional medicine of its day. In that case it, too, it was a reflection of local herblore and folk medicine, reified into a written tradition that imposed constructs from the philosophical tradition. Traces of folk medicine were perpetuated in the written tradition, added to at least in part by Arab medicine and herblore, seen, for example, in some of the plants depicted in the *Tacuinum sanitatis* (Daunay, Janick, and Paris 2009). It is also possible that some aspects of Greek theoretical medicine made it into the oral tradition, perpetuated in folk medicine long after Greco-Roman medicine ceased to be the dominant paradigm (Hand 1976). Folk medicine itself is conservative, but does change over time – perhaps Hildegard's interpretations remained within the oral tradition of the Rhineland well after her death. It would be very difficult to definitively demonstrate her knowledge of traditional remedies given the evidence we have, but we cannot discount Hildegard as a repository of folk medicine and herblore.

One of the difficulties in studying women as healers in the Middle Ages is that their work was not typically recorded, but passed down orally. While this is also the case for men, we have far more written information on men as healers. We would also like to get at the folk culture of the time period, understanding how women were likely repositories of knowledge that served segments of society too poor to afford professional doctors (Ritchey 2014). These same people would be attracted to the religious character of Hildegard's medicine, as Ritchey has shown that saintly female healers' reputations for holiness brought reputations of efficacy to the common people. In the next chapter, we return to the mainstream lineage of Greco-Roman medicine, and examine some of the texts coming after the *Trotula* and Salernitan medicine, especially as they pertain to women.

6 The Legacy of the *Trotula*

Abstract
The *Trotula* went on to influence many medical texts which addressed women's health. Other texts which address diet and health, as well as gynaecology, are examined to trace how the recommendations found the *Trotula* changed over time. In addition, texts in the vernacular became more common, such as Platina's *On Right Pleasure and Good Health,* the *Tacuina sanitatis,* or *The Sykenesse of Wymmen.* Cookbooks also became more common and can indicate some recipes used to treat the ill or infirm. Examination of these texts focuses on dietary advice for women.

Keywords: *Tacuinum sanitatis, Regimine pregnantium,* Platina, Savonarola, *The Sykenesse of Wymmen*, cookbooks

This chapter addresses a number of written sources from which we gain insight into medical recommendations for diet and health after the writing of the *Trotula*. Outside the written tradition, it is much harder to trace the actual health practices and diets of the time. There is much more to diet and health as practiced, of course, than what we find in the written tradition; however, some general trends do emerge. The period of 1250-1450 saw an increase in several literary trends. First, there was a gradual increase in the number of manuscripts written in the vernacular. In the case of the dissemination of the *Trotula* texts, portions made it into other Latin texts, particularly medical miscellanies, where they were combined with fragments of other medical texts. Some extended manuscripts contain, for example, segments of and commentaries on *De secretis mulierum* by Pseudo-Albertus[1]. This text, described in Chapter Three, was less a snapshot of medical knowledge than a polemic in the anti-feminist tradition. Vernacular texts were accessible to a wider array of individuals. While university-trained physicians were

1 Traditionally, this text was attributed to Albertus Magnus, but there is no evidence supporting his authorship.

Vaughan, Theresa A., *Women, Food, and Diet in the Middle Ages: Balancing the Humours.*
Taylor & Francis Group, 2020
DOI: 10.5117/9789462989382_CH06

comfortable reading medical texts in Latin, the vernacular texts could be read by any literate person.

Second, we have the real beginning of the recipe collection or cookbook tradition. These manuscripts are invaluable in helping us understand at least the aristocratic cooking of the time period. While their primary purpose was not necessarily the promotion of a healthful diet, in some cases the manuscripts do contain notations on the properties of the ingredients or the recipes in relation to health. Any person of means would have had access to the advice of a physician, advice personalized to his or her own particular complexion. Dietary recommendations would be implemented (or perhaps ignored, as is so often the case today) by professional cooks expected to be knowledgeable about recipes suitable for different temperaments. Cookbooks, therefore, while perhaps not as reflective of diet as we might hope, do tell us something about health recommendations as well as social class, sometimes gender, and the desire for high-status ingredients, such as spices or game birds.

We begin with a discussion of the *Tacuinum sanitatis*, a book that became popular in the late Middle Ages, likely based on the Arabic text *Taqwim al-Sihha* by Ibn Butlan, offering general advice on living healthfully. It exists in numerous manuscript editions, and was eventually printed in the fifteenth century. It discusses individual food items, and the extant manuscripts and later printed editions are richly illustrated. They were intended specifically for the literate lay audience. While not derived from the *Trotula* texts specifically, they do give us a snapshot of the late medieval interest in diet and health, as well as living properly by addressing all six non-naturals. Next, we discuss the emergence of the cookbook as a literary form. When I speak of emergence here, I do not assert that recipe collections did not exist before this point. In fact, there are recipe collections as far back as ancient Rome[2], but they did not become a popular genre in Europe until the fourteenth century. Third, we discuss some of the direct descendants of the *Trotula*, focusing on a mid-fifteenth century text in Middle English. We'll examine a number of dietary recommendations for women in some depth, looking for similarities to and divergences from the *Trotula* texts.

Tacuinum sanitatis

Beginning in the fourteenth century, new literature derived from medical recommendations began to emerge. These texts, intended not for physicians

2 *De re coquinaria*, attributed to Apicius, circa the first century CE.

but for literate lay people, were known as the *Tacuina sanititis*. The *Tacuinum* exists today in six manuscripts in different collections. The major manuscripts are found in Liège, Paris, Vienna, Rome, and Rouen. The preface to the Rouen manuscript states that the text features six things that are necessary to maintaining health: in effect, Galen's 'six non-naturals'. The first is air, the second food and drink, the third movement and rest, the fourth sleep and wakefulness, the fifth elimination and retention of humours, and the sixth the regulation of emotions. These elements should be balanced, and in medieval belief, God permits good health when the recommendations are followed. The book emphasizes that recommendations would be different depending on the constitution and age of the individual. The author simplifies these subjects, rendering them in tables, because 'the discussions of the sages and the discordances in many different books may bore the reader' (Arano 1976, 6). According to the author, people really only want to know about the benefits of 'science', not all the detail of 'long-winded discourses'. The author then reminds readers that this advice comes from the ancients. This is clearly a work directed towards a literate, non-professional audience.

The sources for the compilation of the *Tacuinum sanitatis* likely came from the herbalist tradition. The original source for all of the various manuscripts may have come from the Po Valley in the late 1300s-early 1400s, or post-plague. Ultimately the source for the herbalist tradition of the *Tacuina* began in Arabic literature with an eleventh-century manuscript known as the *Taqwim al-Sihha bi al-Ashab al- Sitta* (*Rectifying Health by Six Causes*). This guide for healthy living, written by Ibn Butlan, came from a Christian physician from Baghdad who travelled widely in the Middle East (Daunay, Janick, and Paris 2009).

Though most immediately derived from the written Arabic tradition, the source for many of these entries was ancient Greek medicine. The larger part of the text consists of some 280 items on fruits and vegetables, though other non-naturals are also addressed. The therapeutic use of plants has been a cornerstone of both scholarly and traditional medicine almost universally; the *Tacuinum* systematizes that knowledge, focusing on the flora of the Mediterranean region. The first Latin translation of the text was extant by 1266. In fact, the term *Tacuinum* is derived from the Arabic *taqwîm*, meaning tables. The *Tacuina* are abundantly illustrated. The illustrations themselves were copied, as some of the plants depicted did not readily grow in Europe. The depictions of the plants are often idealized (Daunay, Janick, and Paris 2009). There are some mistranslations from the Arabic, as well as some misidentifications.

The Arabic text may have come to Europe through Islamic Spain, as the techniques of herb propagation in the illuminated manuscripts were used in southern Spain. While the *Tacuina* focus heavily on herbs, flowers and fruits, other health advice links the text to the humoral tradition. The book depicts normal living habits, offering simple advice for medical problems, such as eating rice for colic and beets for dandruff (Stoeckle 1984, 707). Each entry focuses on a single item.

Some examples from the *Tacuinum*'s recommendations for the medicinal or health-enhancing use of plants are as follows[3]. Please note that the Church warned people away from aphrodisiacal substances, but they were still extremely popular.

Figure 6.1 Food items and their effects on the body in the Tacuinum

Plant	Specifications	Beneficial effects	Harmful effects
Radishes	fresh from the garden	good for people of all ages, aids urination	may cause flatulence and swelling
Turnips	local white turnips are best	may improve eyesight, possible aphrodisiac	difficult to digest
Carrots	illustration shows purple and yellow varieties[4]	possible aphrodisiac	may slow digestion
Onions	red and white	diuretic properties, aphrodisiac, promote milk production, promote semen production	may cause headaches
Leeks		diuretic properties, possible aphrodisiac, lessen inflammation of the lungs (catarrh)	
Garlic	not too pungent is best	counteracts poisons	harmful to the brain
Kale		ameliorates constipation	may damage the intestines
Lettuce		possible treatment for gonorrhoea, treats insomnia	lessens sexual potency, may harm eyesight
Cucumbers		helpful for fevers (because they are cold and moist), diuretic properties, can thin the blood	may cause stomach aches
Melons	yellow and sweet	good for people with hot complexions, good for people with acute illnesses	may cause stomach aches unless sweetened with sugar

3 All examples taken from (Daunay, Janick, and Paris 2009).

4 Orange varieties of carrots are a relatively recent development.

Plant	Specifications	Beneficial effects[5]	Harmful effects
Watermelons		breaks down kidney and bladder stones, beneficial to the skin, treats fevers, treats cough, treats inflammation, treats urinary tract infections treats hepatitis	may cause diarrhoea
Bottle Gourds		Laxative	
Asparagus		aphrodisiac	
Cowpeas		aids in urination	
Grapes	eaten fresh	cleanses the intestines	
Peaches		alleviates fevers, alleviates stomach aches	
Sour Cherries		settles stomach aches, cures bilious attacks[5]	
Lemons		stimulates the bile, protects against some fevers	
Chestnuts		nutritious, possible aphrodisiac	may cause flatulence, may cause headaches
Hazelnuts		stimulate the brain	may be harmful to the stomach

The items listed above are commonly eaten as foods, rather than strictly taken as medicine. It is striking how many of them possibly stimulate libido or strengthen one's ability to perform the sexual act. While aphrodisiacs have always been of general interest, intercourse and sexual potency were marks of virility and healthy men, and sex was long considered beneficial to women in Greco-Roman medicine. The situation was, of course, more complicated in the teachings of the Church, who viewed the expression of sexuality as a moral issue rather than a medical one. While virginity was the ideal state for Roman Catholic women, the Reformation brought changing views to bear on moral debates. Procreation was a greater imperative in the Early Modern period, especially among Protestants, who rejected the idea of even monastic celibacy. Sexual urges were normal, as long as they were confined to marriage. Thus, the subject of sexual stimulants became more

5 A bilious attack is a collection of symptoms possibly caused by overindulgence in food or drink. Symptoms typically include a headache, abdominal pain, vomiting, and/or constipation.

acceptable even within Protestant religious circles. Outside of religion, of course, aphrodisiacs were always of interest (Evans 2014, 18-19).

While most of the entries do not necessarily mention conditions specific to women, nor do they make recommendations intended for only one gender, the illustrations in the extant manuscripts are notable in that they contain both men and women tending the gardens, harvesting, gathering, or enjoying the edible plants. It is clear this was not a book intended for men only, and that women were certainly as likely as men to benefit from the recommendations and useful properties of the covered plants. While the tradition of herbals is different than the tradition of medical texts, in the *Tacuinum* we see some cross-pollination between the two[6].

Early cookbooks and health guidebooks

The fourteenth century saw the rise of cookbooks as a popular written genre. For some recipe collections, humoral theory is discernible and, if not a direct influence, at least a peripheral one. Some of the early cookbooks contained an eclectic mixture of folk medicine, medicinal use of foods, and eating for the prevention of disease, such as can be found to some extent in the *Tacuinum sanitatis*. Gradually this focus shifted to food preparation for taste, with emphasis on the foods themselves (Thursby 2008, 28). Begun as literature for cooks to the aristocracy, cookbooks gradually became popular for bourgeois households. There is some disagreement among scholars on the first true cookbook of the Middle Ages; there are a number of candidates. They are all preceded, of course, by recipes from much earlier, such as the Roman *De re coquinaria* attributed to Apicius. The following, listed by location, are some of the earliest books classified as cookbooks[7]:

Figure 6.2 A selection of early European cookbooks

Language	Title	Date
French	*Libellus de arte coquinaria*	c. 1300
	Les Enseingnemenz	1306
	Tractatus de modo preparandi et condiendi omni cibaria	1306
	Liber de coquina	1306
	Manuscrit de Sion	1320

6 Pun intended.

7 All text derived from (Marty-Dufaut 2016)

Language	Title	Date
	Le Viandier de Taillevent	1373
	Modus viaticum preparandorum et salsarium	1380-1390
	Le Mesnagier de Paris	1392-1394
	Le Vivendier	1420-1440
English	*The Form of Cury*	1390-1391
Catalan	*Libre de Sent Sovi*	1324
Italian	*Libro de arte coquinaria (Maestro Martino)*	1450
Spanish	*Llibre del coch (Roberto de Nola)*	1477
German	*Buch von gutter Speise*	1350
	Registrum coquine (Johann von Bockenheim)	1430
Savoie	*Du fait de cuisine de maître Chiquart*	1420

In all instances, the early cookbooks are written by or attributed to men, who were professional cooks. It is also possible that they used medical recipes as a model for writing culinary recipes. The first cookbook attributed to a woman is that of Anna Wecker, whose recipes were published posthumously in 1597 (Notaker 2017, 35). Some Early Modern cookbooks also mention that some of the simpler recipes were taken from women cooks. Women, of course, have made up the majority of cooks throughout history, but their cooking was less prestigious, rarely done in an aristocratic household. Women employed as cooks, rather than simply cooking in the home, were hired by households not able to afford a male cook. Nevertheless, women did work as cooks at inns and smaller households, and produced food for sale in the marketplace (Notaker 2017). Their work was not as well-compensated: in France male cooks earned up to three times more.

In the Early Modern period, women did become cookbook authors, and remained so up until the present day. Their books were aimed at other women and household cooks, rather than instruction on the grand cuisine of the aristocracy. In the battle between the sexes, men denigrated women for not having the necessary thoroughness and attention to detail expected of male cooks, and for an unreasonable reluctance to take the good advice of male chefs. By contrast, women often said male cooks were show-offs and spend-thrifts, with no concern for health or economy (Notaker 2017, 21).

Many examples of food recommendations for the ill or weak appear in these early cookbooks. In the Sion manuscript[8], c. 1320, although primarily a cookbook, there are recipes intended specifically for consumption by the sick. For example: *Coulis de poullez* (boiled chicken and sugar), *Eaue rousse de chappon ou de poelle pour malade* (boiled chapon or chicken with saffron),

8 Sion, Archives cantonales du Valais, MS Supersaxo 108 (Kernan 2015).

Choudreau flammen (egg yolks mixed with white wine and verjus), *Gruyan* (wheat and almond milk boiled together), *Coulis de perche* (court bouillon of fish and fresh water, thinned with almond milk), and *Blanc mengier d'ung chappon pour ung malade* (blancmange of chicken for a sick person: almonds, chicken broth, apple and grenadine seeds, and sugar). Most of these recipes are based both on what was believed to be easy on the stomach, and more importantly on humoral theory: balanced, neutral foods, meant for the ill, that could be completely concocted (Gérard-Sai 2012, 97). In fact, blancmange, which existed in various iterations throughout Europe, was one of the most common foods served to women, the ill, and the young with delicate digestions (Milham 1998).

Taillevent (Guillaume Tirel, 1310 – 1395), France's most famous early chef, was employed by both Charles V and Charles VI of France as chief cook and provisioner to the court. A probable member of the haute bourgeoisie, as chief provisioner he would have been literate. A chef was at the time considered rather a lowly, menial profession, but a few stand-outs like Taillevent did earn royal favour and a good reputation. In his position, as was true of other important chefs and provisioners to European royal courts, Taillevent was responsible for providing the proper diet for the royal family. Perhaps the diet was prescribed by a physician, but the chef would also be familiar with the basics of humoral theory and their application to food and cooking, for 'A good cook is half a physician' (Weber 1998, 152). Thus, knowledge of the basics of humoral theory had spread beyond the field of physicians for some time before cookbooks began to appear. Recipe collections were certainly part of literate culture, and perhaps to some degree part of common understanding as well, though this is more difficult to verify.

As mentioned previously, it is difficult to directly access folk beliefs and folk medicine of rural medieval people. Some information can be gleaned from 'church sources, Inquisition records, penitentials, documents concerning the cult of saints, and collections of exempla' (Canadé-Sautman 1992, 92). We know rural and urban folklore interacted regularly, with elements from each side influencing the other. We know traditional medicine was concerned with the conception of male or female children (folk belief contains many ways to predict the sex of an unborn child), and with the safe delivery of a child. These concerns are also common in the work of natural philosophers and physicians, but folk remedies tend to take on a recognizable form. For example, the use of mandragora root to promote conception was gender-specific; certain varieties were thought to be male or female. If the wrong form of the root was used by a man, it was believed he might accidentally become pregnant. Although folk medicine and folk belief were retained and transmitted in the vernacular, some Latin may have been used in the passing on of folk remedies, because Latin may simply have given a folk remedy or procedure an air of authority as it travelled orally from person to person. Prayers or ceremonies to saints might also be used in the service of folk medicine, as well as by the aristocracy, in addition to professionally promoted medicines and recommendations. Midwifery was long the purview of traditionally trained women. Some of their knowledge is clearly part of folk belief: for example, in Salerno, midwives gave women in labour a remedy of seven grains of pepper and a Paternoster[9] that contained a magical incantation, which was condemned by Arnaldus de Villa Nova[10]. However, he praised a similar kind of remedy given to him by a priest. The line between folk medicine and professional medicine was sometimes blurry; sometimes what gave a remedy the cachet of authority was that it came from a person of status, rather than whether it came from a trained physician (Canadé-Sautman 1992).

Considered from Galen's possible influence on folk medicine, we can see connections even into contemporary times. For example, in Latin America, ideas from folk medicine in the twentieth century include the 'theory of "hot" and "cold" diseases, "hot" and "cold" foods, "hot" and "cold" natural conditions, and so on' (Hand 1976, 4). Folklorist Wayland Hand hypothesizes that these beliefs are rudimentary traces of Galen's medicine and humoral theory, taught in academic medicine well into the early modern period. These ideas probably came to the New World with colonists, and continue to survive in a simplified form. Other studies from contemporary scholarship suggest that humoral theory made it into folk medicine of other locations, such as the Netherlands, where a Dr. Bakker kept a detailed record of folk medicine, in which are found traces of the older academic tradition. There may, in fact, be an abundance of elements of academic medicine from the Ancient Greeks leaving their mark on the folk medicine of Europe and the Arab world (Hand 1976).

Perhaps the most striking of the books drawing on an early collection of recipes attributed to Maestro Martino was *De honesta voluptate*, by Bartolomeo Platina (1421-1481, Rome). Platina praises Martino lavishly, but never states which recipes are Martino's and which are his own. Published in the middle of the fifteenth century and translated as *On Right Pleasure and Good Health*, Platina's work combined recipes within a framework of philosophical musings on diet, lifestyle, and health. It made extensive use of the writings of Pliny, as well as Martino. In France, it was accepted mostly

9 Our Father.

10 Arnaldus of Villanova, 1240-1311, physician trained at the medical school in Montpellier.

as a cookbook. As far as we know, Platina had no training as a physician; he simply drew from existing texts for his own guide to diet and health. Platina was a humanist, and he took knowledge of the ancients into his work (Milham 1998). Platina mentions gluttony, condemned by the Church as a sin, as bad for health. According to Bruno Laurioux, 'The vast diffusion of *De honesta voluptate* rested therefore on a quid pro quo: in the book where Platina seemed to reflect on the philosophy of the pleasure of eating, his many readers only really saw it as a cookbook'[11]. (2006b, 537). Platina is sometimes credited as a key figure in the tradition of French and Italian gastronomical writing.

While the field of medieval medicine continued to draw on the Hippocratic and Galenic traditions in the developments of health and diet, medicine became increasingly professionalized. This was also a time of increasing literacy, and general guides on health and diet became more numerous in the late Middle Ages and into the Renaissance. There is some evidence that traditional remedies, or folk medicine, did make their way into dietary recommendations, particularly with food used as medicine. What starts with ancient Greek natural philosophy wends its way through the ancient and medieval world, transforming into fully-formed ideas about how the body processed food, the kinds of food comprising a healthy diet, and how illness could be both caused by improper eating and cured by diet and medicine. A distinction developed between purely medical texts and those more inclined toward natural philosophy. In the guides intended for common use, complicated philosophical discussions were traded for simple ones. Medieval medical texts contain some natural philosophy, but are more oriented around practical treatments. None of this would have been possible without early Greek medicine.

Religion and the body

Thus far, we have not touched on the role religion played in the understanding of nutrition and the body. While the Church largely accepted the theories of Galen and Hippocrates (and to a certain extent Aristotle) regarding the elements of nutrition and the functioning of the body during digestion, it did have quite a lot to say about the dangers of overconsumption, some of which were mentioned previously. The Church controlled a calendar of a

11 'La vaste diffusion du *De honesta voluptate* repose donc sur un quiproquo: là où Platina prétendait réfléchir en philosophie au plaisir de manger, ses nombreux lectures ne virent pour l'essentiel qu'un livre de cuisine'. Translation my own.

great number of fast days, when meat, poultry, and sometimes butter or oil and eggs were forbidden, and also advised eating sparingly for spiritual health. Sometimes Church and medical advice on diet conflicted, and we can see in the development of cookbooks that recipes were offered not just with humoral theory in mind, but also with the Church calendar of feast and fast days. This topic, and the conflicts between the Church, medical recommendations, and actual diets are explored further in Chapter Eight.

Medieval gynaecological texts

Monica Green has traced the history of medieval gynaecological texts derived wholly or in part from the *Trotula* texts through the fifteenth century (2000a). A considerable number of extant manuscripts and incunabula[12] derive from portions of the *Trotula*, often translated into the vernacular and combined with or influenced by other purportedly gynaecological texts, such as *De secretis mulierum*. Such works exist in German, French, Dutch, Italian dialects, Catalan, Hebrew, Irish, and English (Green 2000a, 35). Most contain fragments of one or more of the chapters in the three books of the *Trotula,* rather than the entire text. Some are collections of recipes, such as recipes for pessaries[13], some expound more broadly on female gynaecological health.

A few texts include specific recommendations on diet for women, particularly regarding fertility and conception, along with other information on the non-naturals. Such texts include: *Regimen contra sterilitatem* by Johannes Jacobi (Oxford, Exeter College, MS 35, ca. 1435); *Regimen de conception in complexion flegmatica* by Johannes Pataranus (Jean Pataran ca. 1375-1382, 2 extant mss, Metz Bibliothèque Municipale, MS 282 and BnF MS. Lat. 7066); and *Vorstufe de Frauenbüchleins* (published as *Das Frauenbüchleins* in 1495, by (pseudo-) Ortolf von Bayerland) (Green 2000a, 24).

The Sekenesse of Wymmen

One manuscript directly derived from the legacy of the *Trotula* text(s) is MS BL Sloane 2463 (early fifteenth century), which contains sections of the

12 Incunabula are the earliest printed books, those published before 1501.

13 A pessary is a substance intended to be inserted into the vagina, typically to support the uterus.

Trotula, of Muscio's *Gynaecia* (c. 500 CE) (itself a simplified Latin translation of Soranus' *Gynaecology* [Green 2000a, 21]) and/or sections from *Compendium medicinae* of Gilbertus Anglicus (1180-1250) (Jones 2019), edited together with some noticeable modifications. Written in Middle English, it was translated into modern English by Beryl Rowland (1981). While some of the material in Rowland's introduction has been revised and expanded by later scholars, the translation itself is sound. The Sloane manuscript, according to its own introduction, was written for women to help other women, for they are likely to be too ashamed or embarrassed to confide problems of an intimate nature to men (male physicians being implied):

> Because there are many women who have numerous diverse illnesses – some of them almost fatal – and because they are also ashamed to reveal and tell their distress to any man, I therefore shall write somewhat to cure their illnesses, praying to merciful God to send me grace to write truly to His satisfaction and to the assistance of all women (Rowland 1981, 59).

The author of the text does not make clear his or her gender, but given the time period, when professionalization of medicine by and large excluded women from practicing as physicians, it may have been a male physician writing for the edification of literate women, and perhaps midwives. Unlike the *Trotula*, however, the Sloane manuscript is intended for a lay audience. The *Trotula*, written in Latin, was more likely to have been aimed at a professional, university-educated audience. Following trends in writing over the course of the later Middle Ages, more manuscripts began to be written in the vernacular, meaning their reading would have required some education (and thus would be read by aristocrats or wealthy non-aristocrats), but not the mastery of Latin. While Church services were in Latin, and there is Latin writing in the books of hours[14] that became popular among lay women by the thirteenth century, most did not read or understand all but the most rudimentary of Latin – perhaps the *Paternoster* or *Ave Maria*.

Within the text of this book, entitled *The Sekenesse of Wymmen*, some dietary advice parallels recommendations in the *Trotula*, though with a few modifications. They are presented below. One of the most notable changes is the frequent use of sugar as a medication or as an ingredient in medications. When sugar started to become more widely used in Europe, it was treated as if it had medicinal benefits in and of itself. Certainly, it

14 A book of hours is a small, illustrated devotional guide that was popular by the thirteenth century. It was usually carried by women.

would have also made some medications more palatable (Ziment 2002). Ale is also mentioned more often here than in the *Trotula*, unsurprising given that it was a common and more widely available drink than wine in England. Some of the recommendations come with more explicit humoral explanations than does the *Trotula*. Some are more general, such as the eating of hot or cold foods for certain medical conditions, and some involve specific food recommendations. I have omitted those recommendations intended for the processing of herbs or the making of medicines, of which foods, herbs, or liquids could be key. Instead, the recommendations here are for foods pertaining particularly to diet and health, either to correct humoral imbalance or notable extremes of complexion, or simply to nourish the body properly so the patient gains strength and health.

The concerns in the Sloane manuscript are similar to those of the *Trotula*, and the text is divided by symptom/problem followed by a discussion of possible cures. The conditions addressed include familiar ones such as retention of the menses, excessive menses, 'suffocation of the uterus[15],' 'precipitation of the uterus[16],' 'wind in the uterus[17],' confirming pregnancy, childbearing sicknesses/malpresentations, infertility, and many other issues. Also included are tumours of the breast, thought to be caused by excessive milk. While the terminology is similar, and the manuscript includes some illnesses not recognized today (suffocation of the uterus, wind in the uterus), it does adhere fairly closely to the *Trotula* and the tradition of Greco-Roman medicine.

The connections to diet and humoral theory are still reflective of those found during the Middle Ages, though significant changes to the understanding of the body and its functioning came in the following years (Albala 2012). Adherence to the fundamental ideas of Greco-Roman medicine lasted well beyond the Middle Ages, and would not be seriously challenged until anatomy, chemistry, and advances in lens technology, such as the microscope, moved medicine away from the humoral model. Even after those changes, however, dietary recommendations lagged behind in Europe far beyond when there were medical recommendations for them (Gentilcore

15 Suffocation of the uterus was thought to occur when it detached from its location and moved upwards, placing pressure on the heart and lungs. It also could occur when a noxious substance came from the uterus and moved to the head, where it then pressed downward on the heart (Rowland 1981, 87).

16 Precipitation of the uterus was believed to occur when it fell downwards or sideways. Falling sideways produces side pain; falling downward is now called uterine prolapse (Rowland 1981, 99).

17 Wind in the uterus was believed to come from either external or internal sources, causing it to swell and ache (Rowland 1981,105).

2015). As mentioned previously, Greek understanding of the function of food in the treatment of illness still survives in folk medicine in some areas.

According to *The Sekenesse of Wymmen,* women with access to abundant food and drink, who lived lives of leisure, and who had a relatively 'hot' complexion were apt to have a longer reproductive life. Insufficient food (along with, apparently, too much cogitation) was one possible cause for delay of menses or amenorrhoea:

> Retention of this blood so that they cannot have their purgations occurs in various ways and for various reasons: ... being awake too much, thinking too much, being too angry or too sad, or eating too little (Rowland 1981, 61).

Spicy or pungent food or warmed wine (albeit with herbal additions) could help provoke the menses. The implication here is that an overly cold complexion could be one cause of amenorrhoea. A cold humour could be counteracted with piquant foods such as vinegar or radishes, and here we also see that sweet things like honey were generally considered good for you. The author recommends, after a hot bath with herbs, the woman should drink hot wine boiled with artemisia and eat spicy relishes, such as those made with pepper, mustard, or garlic (Rowland 1981, 67) .

If due to a cold humour, the author suggests processing herbs with vinegar and honey, mixed with water boiled with radishes and madder. Hot baths, especially those augmented with appropriate herbs, were also a means to counteract a cold complexion. Heated baths could aid in a number of bodily symptoms, and we see these prescribed in the *Trotula* as well.

Some of the recommendations in the Sloane manuscript imply that strongly negative emotions could affect the proper functioning of the body. Sadness itself could be caused by a melancholic temperament. Melancholy was associated, in the Hippocratic system, with an overabundance of black bile, considered a cold and dry substance. So, while women's bodies tended to be colder and moister than male bodies according to humoral theory, a cold but dry body could also cause problems for women. While the situation here is not understood in precisely the same way Hippocrates explained it, one can see the link between temperament, diet, and the proper functioning of the body. An antidote to amenorrhoea caused by anger or sorrow (although anger is more closely linked to blood) is to cheer up the patient, have her take baths, and eat good food and drink to build up her blood.

On the other hand, an overabundance of blood could also cause problems, leading to excessive menstrual bleeding or other issues that affected the body negatively. If something caused a paucity of menses while a great quantity of blood was building up, ill health would certainly ensue. Here, as we have seen in the *Trotula* and other sources, eating food that produces minimal blood is a way to ameliorate scant or absent menses. What is explained elsewhere is that women, being colder and moister than men, are often advised to eat food that can be completely concocted, avoiding the excess that could become an oversupply of blood or worse: noxious substances. We have seen this recommendation in the *Trotula* and other earlier medical texts, as well as within Hildegard's *Causae et cure*. Here, however, instead of recommendations for poultry or eggs, the recommendation is for fruit, not typically mentioned earlier in the Middle Ages.

Here again, women with excessive menses are advised to eat food that will 'thicken the blood'. This is in lieu of earlier recommendations to eat food that can be completely concocted. The foods here, however, were recommended for invalids and children in the past: frumenty, rice, almond milk, and goat's milk (Rowland 1981, 79). In fact, they are all white or light-coloured foods, often recommended for those who were ill. Perhaps there was an association with milk, or glutinous substances, but white foods were also associated with refinement. White rice was a high-status food in medieval Europe; white bread, made from highly refined wheat, was also a staple of the elite (Jones 2007).

Within the same section on thickening the blood, there are recommendations for meat. A woman with excessive bleeding is here advised to eat chicken – again, a standard recommendation for food that's easily concocted. We also see the addition here of 'juicy mutton'. Within Islamic cuisine, mutton was considered a 'gentle', easily digested food. However, in the later Shakespearean work *The Taming of the Shrew*, mutton is considered a 'choleric' substance, meaning hot and moist. The fact that this recommendation, from the fifteenth century, is closer to Islamic recommendations shows the continuing influence of the Arab systematists on the Galenic medical tradition, of which the *Trotula* was a part (Rowland 1981, 81).

In natural medicine today, beets are still believed to thin the blood, and beet juice is recommended for athletes to enhance performance with better blood flow (Penn State 2015). They are also considered beneficial in Chinese traditional medicine (Nabinger 2019). This belief may come from the red juice they contain, a watery red substance reminiscent people of blood, thinned or not.

Most gynaecological conditions (as well as non-gynaecological) could be improved by strengthening the body through high quality food and drink. A person who was properly fed and rested was much more likely to be able to cope with any illness or condition, and heal more quickly. For a woman with a weakened constitution, comforting food and drink was recommended. Note the addition of sugar here, at a time when it was more widely available and affordable, and viewed not just as nutritious, but medicinal.

> Have her take comforting food and drink, sugar or roses, poppy syrup, and the juice of mint strained and boiled with a small quantity of sugar to make it sweet (Rowland 1981, 81).

Suffocation of the uterus was mentioned previously; it comes from the idea that the uterus was capable of moving about the female body, that it was not firmly fixed in place. A variety of methods could be used to try to lure the uterus into its proper location, most notably and surprisingly to modern sensibilities, fumigations. Fumigations involved the burning of either sweet-smelling or noxious-smelling substances. If the physician determined the womb had detached and moved upward, the patient was instructed to sit or stand over sweet-smelling smoke, with the theory that the uterus would be attracted to the sweet smell and would move downward, back into its proper place. For a uterus which had 'precipitated', or moved downward, fumigations involved noxious-smelling substances, so the organ might be induced to move upwards and away from the smoke. Other methods of dealing with a wandering uterus are listed both here and in the *Trotula*, and a few involved dietary recommendations. It should also be noted that the uterus was thought to contain corrupt matter, essentially leftovers from incomplete digestion, which could prove dangerous, or 'venomous', as noted here. This is the same belief referenced in the *De secretis mulierum*, in which women were to be feared because the noxious humours of the uterus could poison food or endanger others.

Suffocation of the uterus could cause a variety of symptoms, including pain, shortness of breath, heart issues, and feelings of fullness, as the uterus was assumed to be placing undue pressure on the heart and lungs (Rowland 1981, 87). It could be so dangerous that it could provoke a heart attack, loss of consciousness, or other serious symptoms. While the causes could be numerous, a common remedy involved balancing the humours through baths, wine, or humorally-warming substances. If suffocation of the uterus was caused by a 'bad seed', then the remedy might be dietary as well. A diet intended to strengthen the individual might prove efficacious, provided it avoided foods that might 'increase seed', including egg yolks, fresh meat, pork, male chickens, boar's brains, testicles belonging to strong animals, and finally a variety of fruits, vegetables, and nuts, such as pears, dates and figs, and almonds and turnips fried in honey. Finally, a strong sweet wine, either red or white, and enough sleep should prove useful (Rowland 1981, 95).

One can't help but think that this extended list of remedies for 'bad seed', which causes suffocation of the uterus, is really intended as a list of foods to 'strengthen the seed', or promote fertility. It's possible that these foods also serve as aphrodisiacs, and are associated with illicit sex. To couch this list in a medical treatise overtly intended to deal with women's issues also telegraphs information that might be useful to women, but is not sanctioned by the Church. In contrast to this list, fasting was recommended to destroy the seed, thus making it less likely to cause suffocation. By the sixteenth century, there would also be increasing concern with fertility, decreased population, and the birth of heirs, as discussed previously. It is also possible that this passage is related to that same concern.

'Wind in the uterus' is another condition no longer recognized today. Wind could come from outside or inside the body. Wind from within the body is here understood to come from foods likely to cause flatulence. That same bad air could also blow into the uterus, causing pain or discomfort for women. For wind in the uterus, one could drink wine boiled with dove droppings. Woman with this condition could also abstain from 'windy' foods, 'such as peas, beans, vetches, raw fruits, and raw herbs' (Rowland 1981, 107). Other cures involve ingesting wine boiled with nettle seed or peonies.

Inflammation of the uterus is another recognized condition in the Sloane manuscript. Inflammation might cause pain or swelling. The Sloane manuscript lists no single cause; inflammation might be caused by an excess of either hot or cold humours. The dietary remedies involved ingesting substances to counteract the humoral excess. Humorally cold plants and herbs were recommended for inflammation caused by an excess of heat, while warming plants and sweet things were recommended for an excess of cold humours (Rowland 1981, 117).

For general discomfort after the birth of a child, a plant-based remedy of elderberry shoot juice mixed with eggs and flour, and made into fried cakes was recommended. Fat and egg yolks are warming substances, as is the warmed wine and cumin. These warming substances were probably considered both comforting and humorally warming after childbirth (Rowland 1981, 121).

Various kinds of food and drink are recommended for nausea and incontinence in the Sloane manuscript. In the first case, a woman who can't keep down mead, a fermented honey product, is likely to be pregnant. In the second, roasted tree nuts (hazelnuts and almonds) can be consumed to counteract incontinence, a condition not unique to women, but certainly common after the birth of a child, a history of multiple births, or old age.

A concoction meant for treating nausea in pregnant women should be made with artichokes, salt, madder, chervil, and chickweed mixed with ale. The patient should drink this mixture every morning for three days to take away nausea (Rowland 1981, 163) Note here the use of ale. Many of the recommendations in the Sloane manuscript mention wine, especially as they echo recipes from the *Trotula* tradition or other Mediterranean area authors, but ale was far more commonly found in England (Bennett 1996). This is one instance of modifications made to accommodate local tastes and availability.

A final interesting point, though not strictly relevant to diet in our sense, is the idea that one can favour the birth of a male or female child by consuming the sexual organs of a hare of the opposite gender from the one wished for (Rowland 1981,169). Folk belief is replete with methods of determining the sex of a foetus, and with means to try to conceive one gender or another. This is common in patriarchal societies, and was mentioned previously in a discussion of the work of Michele Savonarola (Marafioti 2010), as well as in the choice of male or female mandrake root. The Sloane manuscript mentions the *Trotula* specifically as a source for these recipes.

Diet is still used in a number of cultures to achieve conception of a specific sex of infant, most often for the purpose of conceiving a male child. Even contemporary scientific studies on diet and sex determination have determined that certain foods – such as potassium-rich cereals – can favour the conception of a male child (Cramer and Lumey 2010). In India, consuming dairy products is believed to promote conception of a girl, while eating sweet foods and avoiding dairy promotes the conception of a boy. In Chinese traditional medicine, consuming alkaline foods is said to promote the conception of a boy. The desire to have a child of a certain sex is ancient, and folk medicine invariably provides remedies, some dietary. This may be one such remedy, as hares are associated with fertility in English folklore.

The *Trotula* text was copied and modified, in whole or in part, for three centuries after it was written. It was a touchpoint of medicine for women, and as it was translated into a number of vernacular languages it became accessible to a greater number of people. Set within the context of emerging interest in health manuals, dietetics, and recipes that combine the interests of diet and health, it gained a wide audience. Even as women were an increasingly small minority of those trained as or allowed to practice as physicians, the reputation of 'Dame Trota' continued long after her name was associated with a group of texts. By the sixteenth century, the influence of the *Trotula* would gradually fade. Yet health guides, especially for lay audiences, became more and more popular. The connection between diet and health would continue, though an understanding of the body would change later in the Early Modern era, moving away from a Hippocratic system. By the nineteenth century, the entire system of humours would be overturned, at least in professional medicine in the West (Gentilcore 2015). It would persist, however, in folk medicine. Further developments in dietary recommendations for women's health after the Middle Ages are explored in Chapter Nine.

7 Women's Diets and Standards of Beauty

Abstract
Looking beyond gynaecological issues, how did standards of beauty affect dietary recommendations, what women ate, and how they presented themselves? Obesity, while viewed differently than it is today, was considered a factor in women's fertility. It was also related the sin of gluttony and other sins which demonstrated a lack of self-mastery of bodily appetites. Examining conduct literature is one way to gain access to cultural expectations of the female body. Religious concerns about self-presentation could also manifest in what has been called "holy anorexia." The anthropology of the body suggest that what women eat and how they look are deeply embedded social constructs which reveal culture attitudes towards gender difference, women, and power.

Keywords: obesity, gluttony, anthropology of the body, bodylore, fertility, conduct literature

Standards of female beauty have been the topic of literature and art for centuries. In our contemporary society, to be a female and to possess a body that is lean and toned, with skin not too light and not too dark, sporting long hair and a youthful appearance is to win the cultural lottery. Those who deviate from the accepted norm are either, at best, invisible to men, or, at worst, ridiculed. Men and women are both complicit in the reinforcement of societal standards of beauty. While the exact ideal body type varies by culture and time period, with a predilection for small or large breasts, narrow or curvy hips, strong or delicate body, light or tanned skin, long hair or short, advertisers and media keep us informed on the latest trends in female body shape and colour and suggest how to change our bodies to fit the ideal.

We also live in a society that, at the moment, is obsessed with thinness. The 'diet industry' makes large sums of money telling us how to eat,

---

Vaughan, Theresa A., *Women, Food, and Diet in the Middle Ages: Balancing the Humours.* Taylor & Francis Group, 2020
DOI: 10.5117/9789462989382_CH07

what to eat, how much to eat, how often to eat, whether one should eat more carbs or fewer, go low-fat or full-fat, whether we should eat 'clean' or concentrate on eating diet foods; keeping up with the latest trends can be about as confusing as keeping up with what our body should be like at any given time. The medical industry is concerned with those who eat far too little – anorexics – and those who eat far too much – the morbidly obese. For those who lie between these two extremes, there is also a host of advice about controlling our cholesterol, keeping fit, and getting to and maintaining the ideal body weight. For those who can afford it, surgery is an option to modify our bodies: to inflate or reduce our breasts, make our noses more appealing, vacuum out excess fat to sculpt our bodies, lift our butts, erase the wrinkles from our faces, and generally improve upon what nature has given us.

Cosmetics

Cosmetics, which have existed for thousands of years, enhance our eyes, rosy our cheeks, even our skin tone, plump and redden our lips, and otherwise work to enhance our beauty to better conform to society's standards. The story of the female body is the story of the social order inscribed upon the flesh. Bodies serve as a symbolic locus of identity, and cosmetics, dress, and other forms of body modification and adornment serve to alter the body to conform to societal standards of beauty. We seek to transform our bodies, and cosmetics are one way to do this. As a symbolic vessel, the female body is a site of social negotiation and control. At any given time, our sense of what is beautiful seems normal and obvious to us, but of course is highly culture-dependant. Cosmetics may be used even when the body itself is largely covered, according to social sanctions or norms.[1]

Recipes for cosmetics have existed since Egyptian times; in fact, the *Trotula,* explored in Chapter Five, contains a treatise on cosmetics: *De ornatu mulierum*[2]. It does not explicitly mention diet, but instead deals with ways to make the skin and hair beautiful, promote soft lips and moisturized skin, remove unwanted hair, make the teeth white, make the skin whiter or both rosy and white, and even outlines several recipes and instructions to tighten

1 While this chapter concentrates on the female body as a locus for cultural standards of beauty, male bodies, of course, are also subject to societal standards of attractiveness and masculinity.

2 *On Women's Cosmetics.*

the vagina to give the illusion of virginity (Green 2002). These directions are given in a straightforward manner (just as the medical recommendations are in the rest of the text), and tell us something about common practice in the port city of Salerno in the thirteenth century. Although a number of other sources seem to point towards light or blond hair as being the ideal of beauty, these recipes present far more instructions for making the hair black, perhaps to cover grey hairs (Green 2002) 'Beauty, though highly subjective, is more than simply a matter of aesthetics or taste. Cultural ideals of beauty are also an index and expression of social values and beliefs – so much so that "the history of [society] is in large measure the history of women's beauty"' (Reischer and Koo 2004, 298). In Salerno, south of Naples on the Italian peninsula, with its cross-section of Christian, Muslim, and Jewish women and Mediterranean atmosphere, it is likely that black was a far more common (and more valued) hair colour than it might have been farther north.

Beauty and morality

Only rarely in contemporary Western society does religion have a role to play in determining beauty standards or our relationship to food. But if one looks beyond the overtly religious reasons to maintain one's health and avoid excess food or drink (the sin of gluttony), there are a variety of ways in which contemporary culture views significant deviation from societal norms of beauty, especially regarding weight, as moral failings. The language of sin may be absent[3] or couched figuratively, but the moral condemnation is still there; just look in the comments section of any internet discussion of diet and weight loss. Some people clearly have a visceral reaction to obese bodies, accusing those who possess them of laziness and lack of self-control (mirroring the sins of sloth and gluttony). Condemnation of obesity also centres around economics: people who are obese are a drain on societal resources and burdens on an overtaxed healthcare system. Obesity is correlated with several chronic diseases, such as Type II diabetes, heart disease, cancer, and hypertension. Obese people are morally faulted for voluntarily causing their own illnesses and using the resources of the health care system. They are faulted for taking up too much room, for not caring more about themselves, for not doing the simple thing – eat less, move more.

The language of moral blame present today is echoed by medieval ecclesiastical writers in the condemnation of sins, sins largely associated

3 Although it is still possible to find it used both directly and indirectly.

with the body. Gluttony was primary among these, for eating too much was a sign of lack of mastery over the body and its appetites. Maintaining incomplete mastery over the body, of giving in to desires of the body, meant the tendency to one sin could lead to others. Gluttony, an overindulgence in an appetite for food or drink, could lead to lust and fornication. After all, if one is willing to overindulge in food, then what is to stop one from overindulging in other bodily appetites? Sloth – or laziness – was also a result of incomplete mastery over the body. In descriptions and illustrations, we see gluttons not just obese but slovenly, lazy, and even lecherous.

Medieval attitudes towards diet and standards of beauty for women are sometimes difficult to ascertain. To begin with, much of the literature focusing on female standards of beauty does not, as is common today, make explicit reference to the size or shape of women's bodies. Descriptions of female beauty might focus on pale or rosy skin, richly coloured hair, sweet breath, sparkling eyes, or other primarily facial features. Descriptions of women who have passed their prime and who are no longer beautiful seem to focus on the quality of their skin, their wrinkles, small eyes, and perhaps a certain tendency towards plumpness, lack of teeth, and warts or other disfigurements. As we shall see, for much of the Middle Ages, there was no specific condemnation for fatness as a hindrance to beauty, and female attractiveness was usually not described in terms of weight. As such, it is hard to relate that period to this in terms of standards of bodily weight or fitness. However, there were dietary recommendations:

> As historians such as Nancy Siraisi and Margaret Pelling have reminded us, attention to the appearance of the body was long considered to be a part of medicine, or at least a legitimate concern for a physician. Indeed, one of the *Trotula* texts and a section of the first English book on midwifery are devoted to cosmetics. The close and overlapping relationships among moral worth, physical attractiveness, and health meant that attending to the body's surface had implications beyond what we think of as 'health' (Fissell 2008, 12).

To explore concepts of diet and beauty in the Middle Ages, we begin with conduct literature, especially works focusing on female beauty – both its benefits and drawbacks. Conduct literature offers a glimpse at competing discourses about the female body, both in terms of beauty and of comportment. For some writers of conduct literature, the most important aspect of female beauty was virtuous behaviour. A virtuous woman's inner beauty would be likely to show upon her face, these authors counselled, making her a natural beauty. For others, female beauty and comportment were a means to cultivate social interactions and improve one's place in society.

Next, we look at a broader medieval system in which the contrast between religious valuing of fasting and lack of concern for beauty contrasted with the secular peasant ideal of food in unlimited quantities and the classic writings of the romances and their descriptions of female beauty. We contrast the medieval valuing of a somewhat plump female body (by today's standard) with a contemporary sociocultural ideal placed on thinness. In both cases, the ideal body type signalled class differences, although the preferred body types have changed over time.

Finally, ideas about agency, health, beauty, and embodiment will help further analyse information available in the Middle Ages. By necessity, contrasts are made both with contemporary Western and non-Western cultures. Please note that comparisons between the Middle Ages and contemporary non-Western cultures are not meant in any way to imply that contemporary peoples from a non-European context are somehow not 'modern' – the contrast is made by way of analogies to different ways of thinking about female bodies and diet. All peoples living today are 'modern', a term that in some uses translates to more advanced, somehow more developed than other peoples. This is a relic of long discredited social evolutionary theory, which arose in the late nineteenth century as part of a wilful misunderstanding of Darwin's evolutionary theory combined with the colonialist worldview and the idea of continuous social 'progress'. The idea was that societies develop from simple to complex, with the pinnacle being the elite of the Western world[4].

Medieval conduct literature

Conduct literature was intended for young men or women to educate them on their duties and social roles. While medieval conduct literature exists for both sexes, conduct literature for women (most often written by men) became increasingly important in the thirteenth and fourteenth centuries, especially in continental Europe. It was sometimes written in the form of a poem, but also appears as handbooks, essays, or miscellanies. One of the best known and most extensive pieces of literature that contained advice

4 Especially, it must be said, the British, who were heavily engaged in both the idea of progress and the colonial enterprise.

for conduct as well as household management for women was the *Ménagier de Paris*[5].

Medieval didactic literature, particularly that of the 'conduct' variety, was a known and apparently popular genre that has received comparatively little scholarly attention. In and of itself, it is a hybrid genre, where one finds a mélange of clerical, aristocratic, and bourgeois texts. Conduct books are, in essence, compendia of known writings pertaining to proper conduct, drawing from the whole of the literate tradition. Intended primarily for the wealthy and those aspiring to the upper middle class, they were frequently copied (and later printed) in whole and in part. The *Ménagier* was one of a number of popular examples published in the late fourteenth and early fifteenth centuries. Other well-known works are the *Livre du Chevalier de la Tour Landry pour l'enseignement de ses filles*[6] from 1372, and Christine de Pizan's *Livre des Trois Vertus*[7] from 1405 (Krueger 2005). An earlier, less well-known work we briefly examine is the *Chastoiement des Dames*[8] written around 1250 and attributed to Robert de Blois. Literature written specifically for women outside of the aristocratic or religious spheres began to appear in the early- to mid-fourteenth century, the earliest popular work being *How the Good Wife Taught her Daughter* (Shuffleton 2008). The audience for *Le Ménagier* likely represents a 'middle culture' as defined by historical anthropologist Jean-Claude Schmitt: '"middle culture" located between the oral culture of the laity and the learned and Latin culture of the clerical intellectual elite' (Schmitt 1998, 381).

While these works were ostensibly written for the instruction of girls and women, bourgeois women were probably not the only intended audience. Such conduct books were also directed at men, as 'part of a strategy for gaining cultural capital in a bourgeois milieu in which men competed with one another on the basis of their wives' obedience' (Epurescu-Pascovici 2012, 220). In such a milieu, a husband was judged on his ability to manage money and political affairs, as well as to manage his wife as she ran the household. Krueger (2005) sees the impetus for many of the conduct books as an imperative to keep household order. An inefficient and unruly wife could destroy the household as much as poor housekeeping. The concern of these authors was order, efficiency, and obedience in the service of maintaining

5 The title of the *Ménagier* is translated into English in a variety of ways: The Goodman of Paris, the Goodman's Guide, or the Good Wife's Guide being common.

6 *Book of the Knight of Landry Tower*

7 *Book of the Three Virtues*

8 *Ladies' Instruction*

social standing. The authors use both exempla and religious teachings to emphasize the importance of wifely obedience and the consequences of disobedience. In the case of the author of the *Ménagier,* did he do this in part to protect his own social standing? He wanted to impress other bourgeois men not only with his erudition, but with his success in demanding an orderly and efficient household. Disobedience on his wife's part might also affect his legacy, as his young wife would no doubt survive him and remarry – it would reflect upon him if his wife was disobedient and lazy, for that would indicate he did not train her well. One could argue censure for poor household management might also lie with her parents, not least her mother, but it would also reflect poorly on the author. The author of the *Ménagier* was no doubt concerned about his reputation even after death.

Along with advice for proper social conduct, some of these works also gave advice on proper self-presentation for women. This presentation could take many forms, but all were recommendations designed essentially to make a good impression on other bourgeois women and men, and, one imagines, to avoid a negative impression as the spouse of an important man seeking upward mobility. Conduct literature itself can be seen as a locus for competing discourses and control of the female body during the medieval period and later (Udry 2002). It can contain both moral statements and beauty advice, presenting a window onto competing expectations for female bodies and souls.

Robert de Blois, author of the *Chastoiement des dames*, writes to teach young women how to behave properly. A woman should, for example, take care to not talk excessively, expose too much of her body, or give off any air of impropriety or unchaste behaviour. He is particularly concerned with vices, such as gluttony, drunkenness, wrath, and pride. These are all common enough subjects for writers concerned with morality, and he cautions that even the least trespass into dangerous areas, such as allowing a man to touch her breast through the fabric of her clothing, will inevitably lead to the great sin of unchaste behaviour (Udry 2002, 92-93). For the reader, Robert seems convinced that the slightest improper touch or gaze on the part of his daughters, and they will have as good as torn off their clothes and hopped into bed with a man.

Interestingly, Robert also offers beauty advice. A woman who wishes to make a good impression must not only know how to comport herself properly, remain chaste, take care not to talk too much, nor to gaze at a man with whom she has no family relationship, but she must also take care to be attractive as well. Here is one of the rare cases where conduct literature offers some direct dietary advice, other than to avoid gluttony. A woman's beauty is described as being apparent in her face most especially[9]. She should be calm and reserved, for anger makes her face ugly. Her skin should have a rosy glow, not overly pale.

> "Dame qui ai paule colour
> Ou qui n'ai mie bone oudor
> Se doit par matin desjuener.
> Bon vins fait face colorer,
> Et qui bien mainjue et bien boit Moillor colour avoir en doit.
> Vos qui mavaise oudor avez,
> Quant vos pais ou mostier prenez, Entretant vos matez en poigne
> De bien retenir vostre aloinne; D'ennis, de fenoil, de cumin
> Vos desjuenez sovant matin (373-384).

> ["A lady who has a pale color, or who does not have a good smell, should eat a meal in the morning. Good wine adds color to the face, and whoever eats well and drinks well should have a better color because of it. You who have foul-smelling breath, take care to hold your breath while you are passing the Peace at church; chew anise, fennel, and cumin frequently in the morning." Translation Udry's (2002, 95)].

Udry notes that the advice given here is not so much to make a woman sexually attractive to men, but rather to make her pleasant in social situations, with inoffensive breath for whomever she may talk to.

In *Le Chevalier de la Tour Landry,* Geoffroy de la Tour Landry also advises his daughters to avoid vice and to give the appearance of chastity[10]. In his work, however, he seems somewhat less concerned about rosy skin. Instead, he focuses on proper posture, avoidance of sins such as pride or gluttony, and rails against 'self-counterfeiting' with cosmetics or other common beauty practices. He recounts exempla in which, for example, God sent the flood because the men and women were overly concerned with ornamentation and *luxuria*[11], thus causing the destruction of most of mankind. He preaches against women who wear fancy headwear, who resembled snails or unicorns, while also expressing outrage at outsized male codpieces. In another exemplum, Geoffroy tells of a man whose wife was deceased, who prayed for a vision of her to be assured she was well. He was

9 Not coincidentally, this is the only part of the female body Robert thought should be visible.
10 As well as, no doubt, to actually be chaste.
11 Luxuria is the sin of lust.

granted the vision, saw demons sticking needles into his wife's forehead and eyebrows, and his wife in great torment. The needles were placed wherever she had plucked her own hair on her forehead or eyebrows[12] (Udry 2002). True beauty, according to Geoffrey, came from within, the result of living a moral and chaste life. This inner beauty would show on the face, whereas sin and vice would make a woman ugly, and cosmetics were inherently sinful because they gave women a counterfeit or false countenance.

In *Le Ménagier de Paris*, there is also an emphasis on wifely obedience. Integral to late medieval discourse on the chastity and uprightness of woman as part of the role their husbands played in bourgeois society, the emphasis in *Le Ménagier* has moved away from the courtly love tradition, in which the love of a women was dangerous and all-consuming. In the haute bourgeoisie, a wife was a form of cultural capital: a chaste and attractive wife who knew how to manage the household well and move through society with grace and charm was a boon, and if the literature is to be believed, a necessity for men hoping to rise in society. Stories told in *Le Ménagier*, such as the story of Griselda, serve to emphasize the necessity of obedience to one's husband. Griselda's beauty is secondary. 'The issue of what women should want and how they are to comport themselves seems fraught with anxiety for *Le Menagier's* avuncular author, the aging husband of a teenaged wife. His book of keeping house is also a book about keeping women – in their place' (Rose 2002, 397). This is accomplished through a number of means, mostly by adapting the stories of other authors as exempla and couching those stories within his own moral instruction. The author also cites scripture and the writings of Church Fathers, such as Tertullian, to underscore his instruction.

While the *Ménagier* is best known today for containing recipes, those recipes were copied from other sources, and contain quite a bit of 'aspirational' cuisine – that is, recipes originally intended for the manor house, some for great feasts, but that could serve as a guide for the bourgeoise housewife to a more esteemed class of cooking, and perhaps enable her or her servant(s) to cook fancier meals for guests. There are no specific dietary recommendations or notes on health, but the guide does contain some similar words about bodily comportment as those seen in the texts mentioned above. For example, as the elderly husband writes to his young wife:

> I wish to speak here a little bit about clothing. About which, my dear, know that if you choose to behave according to my advice, you will consider and pay attention to our status and our means, attiring yourself with

12 The fashion at the time was for high hairlines and absent eyebrows.

respect to the estate of your family and mine, amongst whom you will mingle and dwell each day (Greco and Rose 2009, 57).

The author goes on to explain that his wife must wear fashionable clothes, always presented neatly with nothing out of place, lest she come across as ignorant or slovenly. She should avoid eye contact, walking erectly and modestly. She should look the part of a well-to-do townswoman, mindful of her own reputation and that of her husband.

Medieval ideas of beauty

Another approach to understanding medieval views of female beauty can be found in descriptions of beautiful (and ugly) women. In the extant literature of the twelfth through fifteenth centuries in Western Europe, the written ideal of a beautiful woman is fairly consistent, allowing for regional differences in hair colour, skin colour, and other commonly described features. In a survey of literature from Iberia, Da Soller notes the following example from the *Book of Good Love*[13], which is typical: 'a small head; blond hair; eyebrows set apart, long and arched; a narrow chin; large, prominent, colourful, and shining eyes, with long lashes; small, delicate ears; a long throat; a finely chiselled nose; small, even, sharp and white teeth, close together; red gums; red lips finely-drawn; a small mouth; and her face white, hairless, bright and smooth' (Da Soller 2010, 95). In other sources, Da Soller finds that a trim waist, well-rounded belly, larger hips, fleshy legs, and small feet are also frequently described. Black hair is also noted as beautiful. These descriptions bear similarities to the description of beautiful women from classical literature, and their presence in the medieval literature was at least partly due to imitation of classical Latin literature; however, they also show some individuality and changes over time. The order in which they are described, however, remains constant, showing the importance of the head, then the body (Da Soller 2010). While Da Soller uses this description to compare the ideal medieval beauty to what he posits are evolutionary-based preferences of men for young, attractive, and fertile women, it is also useful as a summary of medieval ideas of female beauty beyond the conduct literature.

Did women have an obligation to maintain their health through diet in the Middle Ages? When we look at the contemporary period, we find a

13 *El libro de buen amor*, attributed to Juan Ruiz, Archpriest of Hita. The first full manuscript was completed in CE 1343.

common belief that it is the moral duty of a woman (or a man for that matter), to maintain a proper body size by eating properly and exercising. In the Middle Ages, food and morality were defined in relation to sin – avoidance of gluttony and sloth – rather than as an obligation to society. However, when framed in the conduct literature, maintaining a pleasing appearance and sweet breath was both a social obligation (at least for members or aspiring members of the higher classes), and a mark of a woman properly trained for adulthood. The equation was somewhat different when placed within the realm of religious belief and outward demonstration of religiosity. This topic is examined in greater detail in Chapter Eight, but a few details are pertinent in the current discussion.

Diet as related to health has been extensively explored in previous chapters. Gluttony was advised against, both for religious reasons, and in the later Middle Ages for health reasons. There was also a well-documented phenomenon involving the inverse of gluttony, what is termed 'holy anorexia'. The goal of eating as little as possible, in extreme cases only existing on communion bread, was one of the hallmarks of female holiness in the Middle Ages. Fasting itself was a common condition approved by the Church for mortification of the flesh, combating lust, and repentance for sins. Some women took it to extremes. Denial of the flesh to the point of starvation was a way to deny the health and abilities of the female body. It was also a way to deny female sexuality. These women were not concerned about their attractiveness to men; they actively sought to make themselves unattractive. St Elizabeth of Hungary, for example, offered to cut off her own nose. Sometimes these women didn't want to marry, and it has been suggested that refusal of food was one way of taking power away from others to control their lives (Bynum 1987).

Obesity

If medieval beauty recommendations concentrated more on the skin and face than on the (covered) body itself, are there clear indications that there was an ideal body type? From the *Roman de la Rose* to *Le Ménagier*, it seems women were supposed to be somewhat plump, with a large posterior, although gross obesity was to be avoided. Paintings and illuminated manuscripts don't make a significant distinction in their portrayal of women. Depictions of very obese women tend to be caricatures (Vigarello 2010, 22). While in some ways the medieval world celebrated the ability to gorge oneself, Christian morality taught that eating and drinking to excess was a sin to be avoided. Still, this does not tell us much about ideals and actual eating behaviour. Up until the late medieval period, for example, for men a large body was considered a symbol of wealth and power. Accordingly, it is possible that a plump female figure was likely a mark of status, at least in younger women. It meant a woman was of sufficient wealth that obtaining food was not a struggle. In addition, some plumpness was a sign of health and fertility.

For older women, however, fatness was a commonly noted condition. A woman who had borne a number of children would no longer have a slim waist. Older women were often portrayed as slovenly and overindulgent, particularly those women we see, perhaps in caricature, as selling ale or wine, serving food, or serving as nursemaids. Sometimes, as in the case of the *Distaff Gospels,* these women are portrayed as overly indulgent in many ways: as oversexed, overfed, prone to drinking, and prone to fatness. If we look at examples of portrayals of alewives, brewsters, and regrators in England during the medieval and early modern periods, such as in the poem 'The Tunning of Eleanor Rummyng' by John Skelton (2011 [1550]), or the portrayals of Betoun the Brewster and Rose the Regrator in William Langdon's *Piers Plowman* (2006), we see these kind of women. The young and beautiful woman, however, seems to avoid this degree of corpulence, at least in stereotypic descriptions; neither was she exceedingly thin.

Vigarello, in *Les metamorphoses du gras: Histoire de l'obésité du Moyen Âge au XXe siècle*[14], looks at descriptions and images of fat people over time. As noted above, there is condemnation of gluttons and gluttony in the Middle Ages. However, he finds no particular condemnation of being fat in and of itself (2010, 26). The moral failure was associated with the act of overeating, and overindulgence in general, rather in the state of being fat. This is in contrast to what we see today, where the state of fatness (as well as overindulgence) is itself a sign of lack of self-control and an indication of moral failure.

In medieval medicine, physicians knew fat was important, but did not describe it as an organ. They thought fat was possibly the result of undirected blood, although fat itself is not the subject of much medical speculation in the Middle Ages. Fat was considered somewhat cold in nature, closest to phlegm in the humours, which it in some ways resembles. Phlegm came from insufficiently cooked blood. 'Phlegm is again the dominant humor in the female body: it makes in it a white complexion, opacity, however blood

14 *The Metamorphosis of Fat: The History of Obesity from the Middle Ages to the 20th Century*

would be the dominant humour in the male body; it makes in it a darker complexion, firmness'[15] (Vigarello 2010, 32).

So, in fact, fat being related to the dominant female humour meant that some degree of fatness in women was considered normal, and the result of the particular humoral make-up of the female body. Whiteness was considered attractive, though a rosy glow was also a sign of health. An overabundance of fat, however, could be a sign of a potentially unhealthy surplus of phlegm. 'A similar picture in Hildegard's writing promised the most irascible gluttons an accumulation of "dangerous and poisonous phlegm"'[16] (Vigarello 2010, 32). One potential explanation for such an accumulation of phlegm was the presence of an 'ill wind' (flatulence). To remedy this situation, there were recommendations for food and techniques to dry out the body.

During the high Middle Ages, attitudes towards fatness begin to change. Fatness comes under critique from several quarters, especially clerks urging self-control and doctors who began to talk about the dangers of fat. We see increased teaching against gluttony. However, the critique does not focus on beauty or attractiveness: 'There was nothing aesthetic about these critiques. Ugliness was not at the heart of the debate. Vice, on the other hand, was central: greed by the subsidence of the body, the graveness of sin before all else'.[17] (Vigarello 2010, 41).

Christine de Pizan was among those writers critiquing fatness, but again as a sign of sin, rather than unattractiveness. By the thirteenth century, doctors were counselling not just what to eat, but how much and how often. This movement for the improvement of health would culminate in the various health guides of the late medieval and early modern period, such as the *Tacuina sanitatis*. Still, these guides emphasize the promotion of good health through humoral balance, rather than strictly the maintenance of an ideal weight or of reducing one's weight.

In general, the female body was described as more vulnerable, more fleshy than the male. According to a source from 1911, it wasn't until the end of the thirteenth century that a trim waist and larger bust was considered beautiful. By the fifteenth century, one can see more awareness of thinness

15 'Le flegme est encore l'humeur dominante du corps féminin: il en fait la blancheur, la densité, alors que le sang sera l'humeur dominante corps masculine; il en fait la <<noirceur>>, la fermeté'. Translation my own.

16 'Image semblable chez Hildegarde de Bingen promettant au plus irascibles gloutons une accumulation de "flegme dangereux et vénéneux"'. Translation my own.

17 'Rien d'esthétique dans ces critiques. La laideur nest pas au coeur du debate. Le vice, en revanche, serait central: l'avidité par l'affaissement du corps, la gravité du péché avant tout chose'. Translation my own.

in artwork (Vigarello 2010, 46-47). This is not to say that standards of beauty did not apply during this time, but that they may have been more focused on other aspects of the female body, such as the face: beautiful skin, and shining eyes.

In the late fifteenth century, we begin to see tight belts and girdles in women's fashion. This may indicate a more conscious emphasis on thinness (Vigarello 2010, 56). Fashions change, however, and it is difficult to tell whether the focus was on thinness, or simply on tighter clothing more apt to reveal the female form.

Medical writers as far back as the ancient Greeks had some concept of obesity as a medical issue. While excessive weight was considered only a symptom of a possible humoral imbalance (for example, insufficient concoction of food leading to the body retaining excess phlegm and fat), they also made clear that for the very fat or fleshy person, movement became difficult, the pulse seemed to become weak, and the person was considered generally unhealthy. In a survey of early modern writers on obesity, Stolberg (2012) notes that Galen and Aristotle, and later Avicenna, each noted the dangers of excess fat. Avicenna, drawing particularly on the work of Galen, noted that excess fat compressed the vessels, and hindered the circulation of warmth, or warm spirits throughout the body. This was in part a humoral explanation, as he saw obesity as due to an excess of phlegm and very cold in nature, leading to possible ill health. In addition, obese people also might not live as long, as they lacked sufficient heat[18]. Giovanni Argenterio (1513-1572, Turin), noted in 1566 that obese women often suffered from infertility. As noted above, though, this condition was recognized in the *Trotula* and as far back as Galen. The French physician Jean Fernel (1497-1558, Montdidier, France), also writing in the early sixteenth century, noted this same phenomenon. Nicolaus Florentinus (d. 1411, Florence), writing in the early fifteenth century, noted that fat women, besides being more likely to be infertile, might be more likely to miscarry or have an unhealthy child. A fat body was one in which the humours were unbalanced, with an excess of coldness possibly leading to further medical issues (Stolberg 2012). As mentioned previously, this was part of a pattern of concern about the impact obesity might have on female fertility during the early modern era (Toulalan 2014).

By contrast, Thomas Erastus of Heidelberg (1524-1583, Aargan, Switzerland), writing in 1580, thought fat could contribute to the heat of the body. He believed fat was a type of waste material, but so was semen and milk,

18 One of the things associated with old age was humoral coldness and dryness, as mentioned in Chapter Two. This weakened the body and made it more vulnerable to ill health.

and so could be useful. He also noted that '[fat] contributed to bodily beauty, by filling out the holes, cavities or crevices between the muscles and other anatomical structures, giving the body a smoother, softer appearance, especially in women' (Stolberg 2012, 372). Was this part of a standard of female beauty that, as we have seen, seemed to favour at least some plumpness in women, enough to give them a soft, rounded appearance? Most early modern authors concluded that the obese person's blood was thick with extra food and drink, and this led to fatness. To counteract this, recommendations ranged from avoiding consuming excess fat to increasing internal heat by eating spicier food, especially by adding condiments that were sour, bitter, sharp, or salty. This is in keeping with humoral theory rather than caloric theory, which would come much later. Other advice included sleeping less, or otherwise warming the body humorally to avoid the excess accumulation of cold humours. Anything warming that promoted the concoction of food was a possible remedy for excess fat. However, this only worked for newly consumed food: once it had solidified to fat in the body, it appeared there was nothing to be done. There was a humoral explanation for why older women became fat: in ceasing to menstruate, the body's method of getting rid of excess waste due to incomplete concoction was eliminated, thus making older women more prone to the accumulation of fatty waste (Stolberg 2012).

Sweating was one means to get rid of excess fat, as it was part of the body's elimination system. Sweat baths were sometimes prescribed in the Early Modern period. Blood-letting was also a possibility, though some cautioned that draining the body of heating blood might exacerbate the problem of cold humours and incomplete concoction. Were the concerns about obesity in late medieval and early modern medical writings a response to changing aesthetics of the body? Possibly not. It is not until the eighteenth and nineteenth centuries that an obese body was described as being aesthetically unacceptable, as the ideal female body became thin, and male body muscular rather than just large. In fact, some medical writers cautioned that obese people might appear to be perfectly healthy, and may even be noted for their pleasing look, but that these looks could be deceiving. It is conceivable that physicians emphasized this point in order to make a name for themselves by devising individual diets for patients who could afford their services. Physician-prescribed diets became increasingly popular in the late medieval and early modern periods.

Medical writing was not always devoid of religious teaching; some medical writing did reflect the religious concern of overeating, or the sin of gluttony. As we move into the Renaissance, Pico della Mirandola (1463-1494, Mirandola, Italy) asserted that human beings were unique creations of God, able to move down the 'Great Chain of Being' to be more like animals, or to strive to perfect themselves to be more in the image of God. This assertion of the unique abilities of humankind may be reflected in the fact that gluttony was linked with animals, and thus also denoted a lack of intelligence similar to that of animals (Stolberg 2012).

Despite medical concerns about significant obesity, some degree of fat was considered pleasing in the Early Modern era, just as it was earlier in the Middle Ages. In reviewing physicians' case stories, Stolberg also notes that only people who were very obese and feeling ill due to obesity seem to have sought medical advice. Those who were moderately obese seemed not to have consulted physicians, and in fact were viewed as having a desirable appearance. 'Some women in particular allegedly even ate very nutritious food on purpose in order to acquire a "juicier" (succulentior) body, which they considered to be beautiful' (Stolberg 2012, 375).

In fact, this lack of concern about what would now be considered overweight or mild obesity may be reflected in the relative dearth of documentation in the early modern period of people seeking treatment specifically for mild obesity. Only when the excess fat caused shortness of breath, lack of mobility, infertility, or other issues was it brought to a doctor's attention.

Since fatness was associated (at least by physicians) with corruption of the body and putrescence (the fat essentially being made up of bodily waste), some physicians noted that fat people, especially women, had a putrid smell. This itself could have been an issue when, for women at least, the existing beauty advice stressed the importance of a pleasantly fragrant odour and how to achieve it to promote gracious social interaction.

There was a difference in the expectations for men's and women's bodies in terms of their degree of fatness. Women, because they were colder in nature, were fatter than men, and were expected to be so. Fat was, in fact, integral to ideas of feminine beauty. Breasts especially were considered essential to female beauty, and a very thin woman was apt to have smaller breasts. In fact, breasts were so important to standards of female beauty that obese men who possessed sagging breasts were deemed to be too feminine, despite their bulk. Very fat women (as well as very thin women), however, were sometimes associated with old age and, by association, ugliness. Older women are portrayed as having large breasts, but they were the sagging breasts of a woman who had nursed children and become plump, not rounded, but sagging and ugly. Men, who were by nature hotter, became feminized through excessive fat and the growth of breasts. They were compared to eunuchs, who also had a tendency to become fat (Stolberg 2012).

It is important to note that, while the points about feminine beauty and diet have been raised here in a general way, there was likely some variation between social classes in terms of aesthetic value, expectations for comportment, and foods women were supposed to consume to maintain their beauty. As previously noted in Chapter Three, those who wrote about food and health (mostly men) recommended somewhat different diets for men and women. Aristocratic women were thought more delicate than peasant women, and thus were encouraged to eat lighter and more digestible food, such as chicken and sweet items which were, by extension, higher status foods. Peasant women were of a courser, if hardier, nature, prone to a ruddy complexion and a constitution appropriate for harder physical labour. A range of lower-status food was recommended for them, when medical writers considered them at all. They didn't need to eat such refined foods. Pork, beef, cheese and rough loaves were adequate for their needs. In artwork, peasant women were also portrayed as being less refined, and at least to modern eyes, less beautiful. Their clothing is plainer, and they lack the white complexions of aristocratic women (Freedman and Marin 1992).

The body as symbol

To reiterate, the body is a locus of symbolic meaning. 'Culture is inscribed on the body. Our beliefs about the body, our perceptions of it and the properties we attribute to it, both symbolic and literal, are socially instructed. ... The way we hold our bodies, the way we move them, the way we accouter them, display our membership in a culture' (Young 1993, xvii). Within the field of anthropology more specifically, there are two primary theoretical orientations in examining the body as socially constructed – the 'body as agent' and the 'body as symbol'. The 'body as agent' approach sees the body as an active participant in the social world. This theoretical approach accompanies a focus on personal agency, or viewing the individual not as a passive cog in the social machine, nor yet a silent and oppressed person for whom we must speak. The 'body as symbol' theoretical approach is common in anthropology and other disciplines. In this view, the body is the site of and vehicle for social meaning (Reischer and Koo 2004, 298).

Female bodies have been subject to socially-constructed standards of beauty throughout much of Western history, though of course male beauty is also subject to social rules and pressures (Marcos-Marín 1999). Women have been the locus of 'beauty work'. The female body is subject to changing social rules about beauty, a receptacle of bodily control. The body also serves as a locus of social control and social discipline. Female standards of beauty have been addressed in multiple disciplines as a system of social control of female bodies and lives, and female bodies as subject to the male gaze. Bodies are also sites for the performance of gender, and both conformity to and rebellion against social norms of gender performance. Mary Douglas was among the earlier scholars analysing the body as metaphor for the society, and the site of action of social symbols. The body itself, according to Douglas, can be read as a text (1996). While that view is now considered overly simplistic, Douglas' work has had far-reaching influence in multiple disciplines. Bodies are also seen to express core cultural values (Reischer and Koo 2004). Bodily adornment is one key way in which to express these values, as are cosmetics, tattooing, scarification, dying of hair, hair styling, clothing, and the shape of the body itself (Shukla 2008).

In another key concept, the body is the location of *habitus*. Originally described by Marcel Mauss and elaborated by Victor Turner, Pierre Bourdieu formulated the consistently used definition. According to Bourdieu, *habitus* consists of 'embodied dispositions created by a process of socialization, that could be seen to structure the socialization of succeeding generations' (Sneath 2018). We embody the structure of the world. Habitus explains regularity without explicit rules, and does not dictate social practice *per se*, but does orient and constrain it. Habitus can include patterns of eating, comportment, and other aspects of embodiment. So, for example, in the conduct literature reviewed above, the emphasis was not just on beauty, but on proper bodily comportment. A woman (especially if she is to be accepted as a member of a certain social class and not be an embarrassment to her husband) should walk erect, with eyes that do not linger on men in any way. Her dress should be neat and fashionable, with nothing out of place, no matter how many layers she must don and keep in place. She should keep her skin clear, white, and soft, and her lips moist and unlined. She should, at least in the medieval and early modern periods, maintain a body that is rounded and healthy, without straying too far into obesity or thinness, as this was considered the most pleasing. To inhabit an acceptable body, one must follow the rules of the symbols and inscriptions that render that body social. One must move properly, eat properly, and conform to standards of beauty.

The emphasis on skin is important. 'Skin materializes as the boundary between the self and the world, the point of articulation of difference between bodies and between body and world' (Young 1993, xvii). In the Middle Ages, female skin was emphasized as a point of contact between the self and society, even more than body morphology. A beautiful woman had clear light skin with a rosy glow. She embodied the glow of youth, and that youth was associated with innocence, purity, and was, at least for the Chevalier de la Tour Landry, associated with piety and virtue. As well, though perhaps less obviously than in the current day, the food women consumed became an integral part of their nature; in fact, it literally affected the humoral composition of their bodies. It could affect the very nature of their bodies, acting as a marker of class. The delicate nature of female bodies required delicate foods, at least in the literature on diet and health. The hierarchy of foods in the medieval world meant that what women consumed was as much of a reification of the social hierarchy as it was a comment upon their gender. Not only were women generally advised to eat more delicate foods than men (especially while pregnant, and conforming to a diet more appropriate for an invalid), but those rules were really only applied to the upper social classes. For the monastic world, as far as we can tell men and woman ate similar, largely vegetarian diets, avoiding the meat that could inflame the passions. For peasants, there was less of a concern with gender-based eating, and more with plenty and scarcity (Payen 1981). That higher classes/castes/social orders use food as a means of distinguishing themselves from lower classes is near universal (Counihan 1999, 8).

While the medieval world was certainly far less fixated on female body shape as a marker of beauty, as well as proper self-discipline, what women ate was to some extent associated with their outer beauty. Proper humoral balance was necessary for the body to function properly and look well. Obesity, not yet the subject of condemnation it would become, was associated by medical authorities with health risks. In Christian morality, an obese body was associated with the sin of gluttony to some degree. Paradoxically, however, it was also associated with age, and the ideal female body of the medieval period boasted a youthful complexion and appearance. More fat was also associated with higher social classes in the sense that food was abundant, and a female body should retain enough fat to be fertile. Resistance to male authority could take the role of refusal of food, and refusal to adhere to societal standards of beauty, a subject explored further in the next chapter.

8 Religious Conflict and Religious Accommodation

Abstract

Church teachings against gluttony and the inherently sinful nature of women may have affected dietary recommendations for health. The virtues of fasting and avoidance of meat were extoled by the Church as a means to control bodily appetites, although a strong anti-feminist tradition in ecclesiastical literature reveals a long-held belief that women by nature were particularly prone to sinful behaviour, as well as tempting men to sin and lust. *De secretis mulierum* will be examined as a particularly egregious example of anti-feminist literature. Other anti-feminist literature, such as the *Distaff Gospels* and some fabliaux will also be examined.

Keywords: gluttony, fasting, anti-feminist writing, *De secretis mulierum*, *Distaff Gospels*, fabliau

As mentioned in previous chapters, the Church had much to say about how the virtues of fasting and meat avoidance contributed to the spiritual health of both men and women. This chapter examines the conflict between recommendations for bodily health and spiritual health, highlighting the sometimes uneasy compromise between medical and ecclesiastical dietary recommendations, particularly for women. The Church regularly condemned gluttony; for some early Church Fathers, it might be the primary sin. Evagrius Ponticus[1] (345-399 CE, Ibora, Turkey) declared around 365 that not just gluttony, but an overt lack of restraint in glorying in fine food was the principle vice left to us by the sins of Adam (Rowley 2006, 79). It showed a lack of self-restraint, and could lead to other, perhaps even more grave, sins. Gluttony was condemned for both men and women, but since women's bodies

1 Evagrius was a Christian monk and ascetic of the fourth century who wrote on a number of topics.

Vaughan, Theresa A., *Women, Food, and Diet in the Middle Ages: Balancing the Humours*. Taylor & Francis Group, 2020
DOI: 10.5117/9789462989382_CH08

were more often associated with sin in and of themselves, rhetorically (at least for the early Church Fathers, going back to the sin of Eve) admonitions to fast and eat sparingly were often directed towards women specifically. Women's bodies were already considered to be polluted, and responsible for tempting men towards sin and pollution. They were also related to unrestrained sexuality. The ancient Greeks are probably responsible for this to some degree, as their medical theorizing found that women, cold by nature, craved the heat of a man through intercourse. When combined with Jewish and Roman attitudes (some the legacy of the ancient Greeks), we sometimes see women portrayed as voracious sexpots, ever tempting men to listen to their bodies rather than their God. By the high Middle Ages in the Roman Catholic Church, priests and both male and female religious were supposed to be celibate. Women presented a constant temptation to sin unless they themselves controlled their appetites as much as possible.

There is a confluence of food, sex, and gender in a number of medieval genres, such as the fabliaux, where the comic portrayals of lustful, gluttonous women were common, eliciting both fear and laughter. While the teachings of the Church may have been considered by medieval lay people, they were most often thwarted and ignored in folklore and literature designed to entertain. An examination of church teachings on fasting will help illuminate female refusal of food as a means of resistance to male control and as a way to claim authority within the context of Christianity and the Church hierarchy.

Medieval folklore and literature are replete with instances of unbridled appetites and the consequences of those appetites. In women, as noted previously, uncontrolled desire for food and sex are often linked. In the literature, many of the women who voraciously consume both food and sex are meant to be comic portrayals, designed to entertain. However, in ecclesiastical literature, consuming an excess of food or sex are both sins, one leading to the other on the slippery slope of damnation. With strict rules about fasting and sexual activity, the Church sought to rein in these twin temptations of the flesh. While both men and women were condemned for gluttony and lust, women were more frequently considered guilty of these sins: part of the anti-feminist tradition in Church writings, but also key to comic depictions of women in folklore and literature.

The female body in medieval literature

The portrayal of alewives is instructive. Alewives, or female brewers (most notably in England, but certainly present in other regions), were key to the production of ale, by far the most common drink in England until the introduction of beer in the later fourteenth century. Ale brewing could be done with relatively little investment in equipment or raw materials. Requiring primarily grains and a cauldron, ale brewing was a household task for many women. In villages, sometimes women would set up a rota, each person brewing on a designated day so individual households would not have to brew as often. In towns, brewing ale could serve as wage work, with ale being sold for consumption out of houses or storefronts. Frequent ale brewing was required because it soured after only a couple of days, hence the constant need for fresh supplies. This stands in contrast to beer, which uses hops as a preservative. The brewing of beer required a more complicated process as well as a greater outlay for proper equipment; it was generally done by men, and eventually displaced female ale brewing by the sixteenth century, as Judith Bennett has demonstrated (Bennett 1996).

A sixteenth century poem by John Skelton called 'The Tunning of Elinor Rummyng' depicts the common link between an alewife and sexuality and relies on familiar comic tropes. Elinor runs a village alehouse, and is herself an elderly and slovenly character who dresses in old clothes intended for a much younger woman. She speaks roughly, is not averse to being paid for sex, and attracts other women to her alehouse of ill repute, so they too may engage in wanton and drunken behaviour (Skelton 2011 [1550]). The poem is written in a style reminiscent of the chant of church liturgy. Elinor is a slovenly old women, wrinkled and ribald, affecting a more youthful guise as she spends her days both inebriated and encouraging inebriation in others; she is the culmination of several centuries of less than flattering portrayals of alewives. Alewives were often portrayed as sinful temptresses, luring others into drunkenness. There were implications of prostitution and perhaps witchcraft in their portrayals (Bennett 1996; Vaughan 2011). As for Elinor:

She is somewhat sage
And well worn in age:
For her visage
It would assuage
A man's courage.
Droopy and drowsy,
Scurvy and lowsy,
Her face all bowsy,
Comely crinkled,
Wondrously wrinkled

Like a roast pigs' ear,
Bristled with hair.
...
And yet she will jet
Like a jollivet,
In her furrèd flocket,
And grey russet rocket,
With simper and cocket
(Skelton 2011 [1550]).

In this caricature used for comic effect, a wrinkled old woman is compared with a pig's ear, hair still attached, after roasting. She is well past her prime, yet wears the clothes of a much younger woman and flirts with men. In illustrations of Skelton's poem, she is fat, wrinkled, drunk, altogether unattractive and sinful, and her portrayal is much like others of drunken or gluttonous figures used to illustrate the opposite of proper behaviour.

This figure of an older woman, a slave to her appetites and both a dangerous and laughable figure, appears in a number of other types of literature. For example, in the fifteenth century book *The Distaff Gospels*, or *Les Évangiles des Quenouilles* (wildly popular, with multiple printings and translations into multiple languages), previously discussed. In the *Distaff Gospels,* some remedies for various problems, such as for husbands who don't have sex frequently enough, are recorded in the Gospels. For example, one of the women proclaims that giving catnip to one's husband or lover will provoke his sexual appetite. In response: 'This is true', said Burghe Fauvele, 'because I did that with my husband and I prepared a salad with it. But that love lasted only six weeks and this is why I think that it must be repeated often' (Garay and Jeay 2006, 103).

As the women speak to each other on these successive nights, we see a parade of caricatures of dubious women who behave in ways unsanctioned by society or good taste. These characters include Dame Ysengrine du Glay (Ysengrine the Joyous), a 65 year-old midwife who has not just been married five times, but has taken several lovers to boot. She is married to a much younger husband and is worried he will be unfaithful. Another woman of dubious character is Transeline du Croq (Transeline the Hooker), age 60, skilled at divination and the concubine of a priest. Abonde du Four (Abonde of the Oven) is an obese retired prostitute. Sebile des Mares (Sibyl of the Swamps), age 57, is from Vaud, the origin of the Waldensian Heresy. She is associated with heresy and witchcraft. Gomberde la Faee (Gomberde the Sorceress) is not getting nearly as much sex as she wants from her husband.

Marotte Ridee literally means 'Marotte the wrinkled'. Finally, Berthe de Corne (Berthe the Horny), is about 80 and secretly trained in medicine by her father, a doctor, implying that she practices medicine illegally (Vaughan 2014).

The characters in *The Distaff Gospels* fit the comic trope of oversexed old women. They are associated with prostitution, witchcraft, and dubious medicine. They are described as obese or thin as a rail, and none are attractive. They engage or have engaged in professions condemned by the Church, and none are paragons of virtue. Nor, it must be said, were many people of the aristocracy, but upending expectations of Christian behaviour brings comic pleasure. We can also see that, in part, this portrayal was class-based: lower class women were judged to have less self-control, and thus were more likely to be gluttons or in pursuit of sexual pleasure, at least in the genres presented so far. Since this was a book written for the literate – perhaps the Burgundian court – amusing portrayals of peasant women would have elicited laughter. We will see this is not necessarily the case in the loathly lady tales or the fabliaux.

In the *Distaff Gospels,* another example of using food to enhance the sexual desire of the man[2] is found in Chapter 18. If someone has a cock that is slow and shy, the woman should rub his crest with garlic, and he will perform his duties with the hens. In response: 'If someone could find the herb which revives shy husbands', said Marotte Ridee, 'I would give my shirt and even beg for my bread' (Garay and Jeay 2006, 151). The women of the *Distaff Gospels* may be old, lewd, and craving both sex and independence from their husbands, but the book itself does not exclusively mock them and their 'gospels'; it also gives them voices and shows their concerns. This is perhaps a modern reading of the tale, but in some ways is akin to Chaucer's portrayal of the Wife of Bath – an argumentative, bossy, difficult woman who has had multiple husbands. Comedy is evident in her portrayal, but Chaucer also portrays her as, fundamentally, a woman who wants some say in her marriages and in her life.

Another take on ugly women, sex, and food present in medieval literature is the 'loathly lady' tale. These tales are found primarily in Ireland and England. Perhaps the most famous tale of the genre is that of the Wife of Bath: we see her independent streak, but she is ultimately tamed by the love or instruction of a man. Examples of the loathly lady tale type can be found in some early Irish tales, and she also makes her way into Gower and

2 The medieval comic trope of the cuckolded husband or impotent man was considered just as amusing as an ugly, gluttonous, or oversexed woman.

Spencer, among others (Passmore and Carter 2007). She has large appetites, most notably for food and sex. She is sometimes like a beast, sometimes merely a woman writ large, unashamed of her physicality or her appetites. Her insatiable desires make her revolting in appearance, or at minimum unattractive and fleshy. However, there is a tendency in loathly lady tales for rewards to come to men who can get past their fear and revulsion and approach the loathly lady as a lover. Sometimes men are rewarded with a beautiful woman, the transformation often effected when the husband of the loathly lady, usually married to her under duress, decides to have sex with his wife despite her appearance. Sometimes, as in the Wife of Bath, the man might be rewarded with a different kind of relationship, one in which the woman has more power than was customary, but that nonetheless brings the reward of a true partnership (Rigby 2000).

In the tale of Sir Gawain and Lady Ragnelle, King Arthur's life is threatened unless he learns the secret of what women want. Ragnelle reveals this secret to King Arthur on the condition that she, a fleshy, beastly creature, be able to marry Sir Gawain. Her answer, that women want 'sovereignty', the ability to make decisions about their own lives, is the correct one. Arthur's life is saved, and Gawain marries Ragnelle. Ragnelle is portrayed almost as a monster; with huge claws, she tears into her food, eating enough for six men. When Gawain dutifully goes to bed with her, she suddenly changes into the most beautiful woman he has ever seen. According to Susan Carter:

> Dainty and selfless eating is a signal of femininity; not only do women allow men the privilege of speech at a dinner date, they also surrender the best food, and eat less than men while nonetheless listening attentively and sympathetically ... Ragnelle ripping into enough food for six with her three inch long talons breaks the codified rules as emphatically as she transgresses the conventions of beauty (Carter 2001, 148-149).

In yet another genre, the fabliau[3] at first glance appears to be anti-feminist: women are usually oversexed and adept at finding ways to take lovers. The conclusion of quite a few fabliaux is a reminder that women must obey their husbands and remain faithful: if they do not, significant punishment may be

3 A fabliau (pl. fabliaux) is a comic tale performed by jongleurs in northeastern France, primarily in the thirteenth and fourteenth centuries. They are frequently mildly obscene, with sexual and scatological themes being common. They were sufficiently widely known to have been reworked by Boccaccio and Chaucer and appear in *The Decameron* and *The Canterbury Tales*.

meted out, up to and including brutal beatings. Women often do not come out well in the fabliaux; on the other hand, neither do men. However, a more complete reading of the fabliau corpus shows that women are often smart, cunning, and successful at getting what they desire. Men of the fabliaux are frequently dim, overly trusting, or greedy. Here we see women with agency and skill, though these are not always put to socially sanctioned use. Anti-feminist elements are certainly present, but one must also attend to the whole picture (Chatten 2002).

Food consumption is often part of the fabliaux. Feasting is described in both oral and written literature of the Middle Ages, especially in epics, but ritual feasting is almost always depicted as integral to aristocratic life, attesting to the generosity and power of the host (Schulman 2007). On the other hand, ecclesiastical literature condemns gluttony and, as we have seen, links it to sexual excess. In fact, this link between food and sex is often on display in the fabliaux, although to comic effect rather than as a warning against sinful behaviour (Gordon 2008). Cuckolded husbands have wives who gift sexual favours as well as the best of the larder to their lovers[4]. The use of food as a metaphor for sexual organs is also in evidence – sausages and nuts abound in the language of the fabliau:

> Fabliau characters are what they eat, morally and socially. In the fabliau, as in real life, food habits and food symbols can be an indication not only of identity but of morality. Moreover, a person's relations to food, or what one eats and how it is eaten, is an indication of character. This relationship between morality and food is the basis for most of the culinary comedy in the fabliaux (Gordon, 2007,108).

In 'The Priest and the Woman'[5] (Dubin 2013) we meet a wealthy and fashionable city woman who invites a priest to be her lover while her husband is out of town. She has her servant prepare a meal and a bath for the priest to welcome him warmly. The serving girl prepares 'peppered pasties, meat in a pot, and good clear wholesome wine' (lines 21-22).

Here we have good wine, probably expensive, along with two kinds of meat, one in the pasty with pepper, and another boiled. After her husband arrives unexpectedly, she tricks him into believing the priest just stopped by and is about to leave with his pasties. The husband insists on providing

4 See, for example, 'The Cleric Behind the Chest' ('Le cleric qui fu repus derier l'escrin') (Dubin 2013).

5 "Le prestre et la dame".

his hospitality, and the table is set with elegant cloth and candlesticks for the three of them. The wife deliberately gets her husband drunk on wine while they eat abundantly.

> They cut the pasties up and break
> them, and the priest and woman make
> an effort to pour lots of wine
> until they've given, by design,
> him so much alcohol to drink
> and peppered pies, beyond the brink
> of total drunkenness has passed
> the master of the house (lines 97-104).

The husband then goes on to brag that he has a thousand pounds stashed away, tries to impress the priest by speaking Latin, German, and two Dutch dialects (badly), and boasts of his accomplishments and largesse. The wife uses food and drink both to entice her lover, and to render her husband too drunk and addled to realize he is a cuckold. The sin of fornication here is not condemned, but rather her husband's susceptibility to gluttony and drunkenness are a sign of his weaker mind. Such is the subversion found in the fabliaux.

In all of these genres, overindulgence in food is related to bad behaviour but also to power, especially for women. On one hand, the Church teaches that female sexuality, like female eating, needs to be restrained and controlled. Some early Church fathers, such as Jerome, advocated abstinence and restraint for all Christians, but were especially concerned about the innate sinfulness of women. They advocated regular and stringent fasting for women as perhaps the best means for women to have at least some control over their sinful natures. Gluttony inflamed the passions, and increased the likelihood of committing sexual sins. To be clear, these writers also recommended fasting for men, but the benefits for women were most clearly directed towards taking control of their sexual natures, as they were thought to be too morally weak for self-control (Grimm 1996).

We can assume that lay medieval people had a much more ambivalent attitude towards gender, food, and sexuality. Within the comic tales of the fabliaux, women can use food to dupe men and to demonstrate their own cleverness. Depictions of the alewife, meant for comic effect, warn about the dangers of loose women, drink, and dishonesty. On the other hand, they also show women with some power, owning or running businesses, providing services that are much in demand. The use of food renders these women powerful. The loathly lady tales also contrast beauty and ugliness, appetite and restraint as an anxious expression of the benefits and drawbacks of female power. Women take on some of the attributes of men – powerful, hungry, formidable adversaries – who, in the end, want control over their own lives, just as men do.

In each of these genres, women's engagement with food and drink are used to challenge typical gender roles. They are also used to challenge church teachings. In them, authors sometimes express derision towards women who overindulge in fleshy pursuits, and towards the men who are unable to control them. Food and sex are linked. Transgressing social norms and female power are linked. However entertaining medieval people found these stories[6], it is clear that medieval women expressing power through consumption of food and drink, or using food and drink to intimidate or lure men so they could be more effectively controlled, were tropes that were meaningful and understood by the reader or listener, even if only used to comic effect.

Food, sexuality, and religion

This relationship between the stomach and the sexual organs was nothing new in the context of Christianity. In fact, it predated Christianity, as the early Church fathers drew upon both Jewish culinary thought and Roman culinary philosophy in their own condemnation of eating to excess. Stoic philosophy, the Hellenistic school of thought especially popular among Romans, placed an emphasis on natural appetite and plain food in its culinary recommendations. Stoics eschewed sauces, sweets, appetizers, and other foods that were both luxurious and intended to artificially provoke the appetite. They also linked the human appetites – for both food and sex – and urged a moderate approach that would artificially enflame neither. Western Christianity in its foundational forms was also influenced by the ascetic and eremitic movements of the East, especially in Egypt and other areas influenced by Eastern Christianity. Adherents to this ascetic movement believed meat and wine provoked lustful urges. Those taking this viewpoint to the extreme moved to the desert to undertake solitary and/or ascetic lifestyles, which typically included rigorous fasting, avoidance of meat and wine, and consumption of raw food, all in an effort to control sexual desire (Laudun 2013).

6 The audiences here would have been wealthy and/or aristocratic and literate.

Stoic dietary theory was one of the foundations of the simple communal meal that became part of Christianity as it grew in influence, with bread and wine at its centre. Simple foods, presented without elaborate spices or sauces, were not only the source of Stoic meals, but also became the communal meals of the religious. Ideally, no meat was included, and repasts remained simple. It is not surprising then that the Church drew from this tradition when emphasizing the dangers of gluttony. Stoic philosophy was also apparent in the abundance of 'fast days' on the Christian calendar, in some places and at certain time periods making up half or more of the calendar. Fast days were days when, at a minimum, no mammalian or avian flesh was eaten, though fish was permitted. Very few foods were actually forbidden outright in Christianity. The impetus for this change from the strict Jewish dietary laws of the earliest followers of Jesus to a philosophy that declared all things are made by God, and therefore no food is forbidden, was rooted in the decision to accept Gentile members into the Jesus movement. Paul, especially, seems to have been an advocate for this strategy. Early converts, members of the Roman Empire, would have had regional dietary habits based on Roman cuisine. "Fast days" were, therefore, not based on Jewish dietary laws, but instead on the avoidance of food that might enflame the passions, leading one potentially into sin. In practice, and largely in accordance with humoral theory, meat, generally humorally hot in nature, was forbidden on fast days, while fish, humorally cold in nature, was permitted. The correspondence is not one to one, as Christian dietary guidelines imperfectly match humoral theory, but there are concordances between the two. It is possible that humoral theory, which likely informed Stoic philosophy to some extent, had more than just a passing influence on Christian dietary regulations. Fasting cycles themselves may have come from Greco-Roman medical advice that suggested engaging in short periods of fasting on a seasonal basis to prepare the body for a new season. As demonstrated in Chapter Two, humoral theory became associated with seasons (as well as directions, colours, life stages, and other features). The writings of Galen do not emphasize this connection, but it is implicit in his work. The Christian church may have woven together Greco-Roman advice with ideas about purging sin and glorifying the suffering of Christ (van Winter 2007, 57-58).

A fast day might also forbid the consumption of any animal product, such as eggs, butter, or cheese. The strictest and longest fasts occurred during Advent and Lent, while regular fasts took place every Wednesday and Friday, and sometimes Saturdays as well (van Winter 2007, 30). Technically 'fast' days were days of abstention: to abstain from the consumption of animals or animal products. There were also days involving a true fast – the eating of less food and fewer meals[7]. For much of the Middle Ages, most people, unless engaged in heavy outdoor labour, ate two meals per day if they had the means. During a true fast, they might only eat one meal per day. Men and women religious often strove to engage in this kind of fast on a regular basis, sometimes restricting themselves to bread, water, and some vegetables. A common penance involved a certain number of days of consumption of coarse bread and water, with perhaps green herbs for flavour (Carlin and Rosenthal 1998, 12). The idea here was to engage in the mortification of the flesh, not just in atonement for sins, but also in an effort at self-mastery and avoidance of future sin, possibly provoked by consuming rich food.

If one were wealthy, an elaborate style of cuisine developed in which fast days were observed to the letter of the law, but not exactly in spirit. Whole menus were developed and recipes created to make the diner feel he or she was consuming forbidden food. Methods included doctoring fish to look like other meats, using almond milk in place of cow's milk, using various natural food dyes to change the appearance of food, and otherwise imitating the look, if not the taste, of feast day dishes. Lent might be spent eating delectable fresh fish, stocked in ponds on wealthy estates, or carted in from nearby streams or oceans, eating concoctions of fruit and ground nuts, and generally avoiding feeling the lack of meat, milk, and eggs. The wealthy might even pay someone else to fast for them (Carlin and Rosenthal 1998). For the average person, however, fast days generally meant vegetables, plain bread, and perhaps dried, smoked, or salted fish[8]. Anyone who has ever eaten stockfish[9] or salted fish can testify to the fact that, while these substances do have their own peculiar charms, one quickly tires of them if eaten regularly. For most people, fresh fish was prohibitively expensive unless they lived near a large body of water or river. Even wealthy abbeys were sometimes criticized for cuisine that strayed too far into the realm of elite dining. The Cluniac reforms[10] were, at least in part, undertaken to address the excesses of the table present in some religious communities.

7 Fast and feast day customs did vary from place to place, and were not uniform throughout the Middle Ages. The rules cited here were common in Western Europe.

8 Most people did not live near enough to large water sources for regular access to fresh fish. Multiple methods of fish preservation developed, and those who could not afford fresh were relegated to eating preserved fish or doing without.

9 Stockfish was dried fish, usually cod, which in its desiccated form was extremely hard, if long-lasting. It required soaking and boiling to become edible.

10 Cluny, a Benedictine abbey in eastern France, became the site of a movement to return to stricter adherence to the Benedictine rule beginning in the tenth century.

Sumptuary laws were enacted to try to prevent common folk from being able to purchase spices or other items to make too elaborate a cuisine, although such laws were often laxly enforced or ignored.

Women, as we have seen above, were often linked to both food and sexuality. As such, they were sometimes advised to fast stringently to avoid their own sinful natures and the possibility of inflaming the passions of men. Tertullian, famously, wrote against any female attempt (present most strongly, he believed, among gentiles) to show her beauty, or enhance it with hair dye, cosmetics, or fancy clothing:

> But why are we a (source of) danger to our neighbour? Why do we import concupiscence into our neighbour? Which concupiscence, if God, in *'amplifying the law',* does not dissociate in (the way of) penalty from the actual commission of fornication, I know not whether He allows impunity to him who has been the cause of perdition to some other ... Are we to paint ourselves out that our neighbours may perish? (Tertullian 2017 [1885])

This attitude became commonplace in ecclesiastical writing. It is seen, as outlined in Chapter Three, in the *De secretis mulierum*. Pope Innocent III (r. 1198-1216) also addressed the subject of women and gluttony. When misogyny becomes combined with advice on the sin of gluttony, we can see where some of the condemnation of women comes from. For example:

> Gluttony demands a costly tribute, but it returns the smallest value, because the more delicate the foods are, the more stinking the excrements are. ... Gluttony closed paradise, sold the birthright, handed the baker, beheaded the Baptist. ... 'For the lips of a harlot are like a honeycomb dropping, and her throat is smoother than oil; but her end is as bitter as wormwood and sharp as a two-edged sword' (Albala 2014, 280-281).

Women were a source of sin, placing not only their own mortal souls in danger, but potentially the souls of men as well. Any inflammation of the appetites could lead to overwhelming temptation to sin, through gluttony, sloth, drunkenness, and fornication. A woman who didn't control what she ate or drank might be in danger of unchaste behaviour, or of losing her virginity. Ambrose (337-397 CE), the noted theologian, remarked that Judith's fasting and temperance allowed her to defeat the drunken Holofernes and his equally drunken army (Carlin and Rosenthal 1998, 12). The contrast of the holy and simple eucharistic meal of bread and wine with images of sin and gluttony is also illustrative of the contrast between fast and feast, or grain and flesh. Potentially, this could be correlated with a contrast in gender associations – male versus female – although male gluttony was also condemned. In the *Canterbury Tales*, Elizabeth Biebel notes:

> The high-protein content of meat has contributed to the traditional view that meat is the appropriate food source for men. Conversely, women have been aligned both with vegetation and with butchered animals. While the nurturing, gentle, and other so-called feminine qualities are seen as being reflected in plant life, woman's physical attractiveness to heterosexual man is at time described in meat-like terms (Biebel 1998, 16).

Chaucer, claims Biebel, extends this metaphor when he writes about the differences between women and men in the *Canterbury Tales.*

Consequences of overindulgence

If we take the medical view, doctors themselves advised against overindulgence and recommended eating according to humoral type. We certainly see, from the texts examined previously, that medieval people associated women with sexuality, food preparation, and gluttony. However, what evidence do we have that people actually followed the diets doctors prescribed? In addition, do we know how seriously medieval people took the ecclesiastical admonishments against gluttony, and obedience to Church rules about fasting? We know both teachings exist in written form, and were extolled by their respective advocates, but how much did they interfere with daily life? If women were associated with gluttony, fornication, and sin in the written tradition, was the same true in the course of everyday life? For peasants, especially, did the exigencies of daily living and the necessity of growing, processing, or purchasing food outweigh any health recommendations or Church teachings?

Food supply was, especially in times of scarcity, probably the major determinant as to what people ate. There is certainly reasonable evidence that Christian medieval people followed the rules of fasting to some considerable degree. The number of recipes for fast days in the recipe collections and cookbooks that began to appear in the 1300s, even if they were intended primarily for aristocratic audiences, certainly bears that out. Evidence suggests this was the case for most people. For example, stable isotope analysis from several late medieval burial sites in northern England suggests that townspeople consumed much cereal grain (likely in the form of bread or pottage, frumenty, and other common dishes), but also seemed to have consumed quantities of pork and fish, most likely freshwater eel and marine fish. The sites chosen were socially diverse, suggesting that basic guidelines of fast and feast days were generally followed by the population of all social classes (Müldner and Richards 2005).

Evidence for fasting exists in other sources as well. Many ecclesiastical traditions make much of the religious duty of fasting, outlining the reasons for fasting and its importance, and insisting on the proper dates for fasting. As there was some variation in the 'Ember weeks', or weeks outside of Lent when one must undertake a great fast, there was some tension around what those dates should be. In one example, 'Seasons for Fasting', an Old English poem in the sermon and vernacular complaint traditions, urges people to follow the local rules. It was aimed at priests in particular, but shows how ingrained fasting was in the Christian calendar (Hilton 1986). There is also evidence that observing periods of fasting was considered one of the minimal requirements for Christian life (Tanner and Watson 2006). Works of art, such as *The Fight Between Carnival and Lent*, the sixteenth century work by Pieter Bruegel the Elder, includes the typical foods of Carnival and of Lent in the Low Countries. On the Carnival side of the painting, we see pork chops, eggs, waffles, and people drunk on alcohol, as emptied tankards lie on their sides. On the Lenten side there are fish, greens, water to drink, and pretzels.

Putting aside for a moment the question of whether or not people followed medical advice, an exploration of the idea of women's relationship with food within the religious context is instructive. We have already seen that women were linked with food and sin, but also with food and nourishment. Women's work to provide food for the family is a noted cross-cultural phenomenon, and until recently was a given in most societies (Cairns and Johnston 2015). Is it any wonder that, given these two strong and opposing cultural undercurrents, women were moved in the direction of refusing food to make a statement about themselves and religious belief, or themselves, social expectations, and social control of their bodies?

Women and fasting

In the 1980s, several authors wrote about the phenomenon of 'holy anorexia[11]', the refusal of food within the context of an assertion of holiness and religious

11 Also known as 'anorexia mirabilis'.

identity. The phenomenon was found in greater numbers among women from the thirteenth to the sixteenth centuries, and was a part of the hagiography of some female saints, including Catherine of Siena. Extreme deprivation of food and drink among men was typically limited to hermits, men who retreated into the desert or other areas where they could largely avoid contact with the world (Bynum 1985). Holy anorexia has been interpreted in various ways, but a feminist interpretation understands these women to have been working within a cultural and religious system by exercising agency and using the body as a locus of resistance and power where there were few other available options. Hildegard of Bingen, for example, was sometimes forced into the narrative of the suffering holy woman, and her illnesses may have been exaggerated in order to make her claims and goals more palatable to Church leaders. She was not permitted to be solely a strong and intelligent theologian, she had to fit into the acceptable female tropes of holiness and religiosity.

Stories of women who subsisted only on the Eucharistic host, the most extreme form of holy anorexia, far outnumbered the stories of men who followed fasting to this extent (hermits alike) during the Middle Ages.[12] Women also reported religious visions or miracles associated with the Eucharist far more frequently than men. Such stories might involve, for example, the host turning to honey or meat in the mouth of a woman. Even before the doctrine of transubstantiation was adopted at the Fourth Lateran Council in 1215, the Church promoted the view that the essence of the Eucharistic meal – bread and wine – turned to the literal body and blood of Christ after consecration. The visionary Julian of Norwich (1342-1416) saw Christ in his symbolic capacity of a mother, feeding the faithful with his own body. The Eucharistic meal was central to Christian identity and practice as few other things were. The miracles of the host turning to another, higher status, food in the mouths of recipients served to underline the bread and wine as fortifying meals – spiritually fortifying, but with a nourishment far beyond that of simple bread.

Exempla, or tales used to teach Christian morality and behaviour, are far more likely to involve food when they are about women, particularly fasting, abstinence, and receiving of the Eucharist. Though they represent the central character in far fewer exempla than men, approximately 50% of the stories of women involved food (Bynum 1985, 4). One such story is that of Lidwina of Schiedam (1380-1433), pious from a young age. In her case,

12 Bynum reports thirty cases of women to one or possibly two cases of men during this period (Bynum 1985, 3).

illness was most often associated with fasting, sometimes to extremes. After a fall that left her mostly paralyzed, Lidwina took in less and less food until she finally stopped eating altogether. It is possible that she used illness and fasting to resist control by others. She framed her suffering, however, as an exercise in piety, and influenced others to follow her example, including her nephew, whom she prayed would get ill so he could understand redemptive suffering, and a hermit named Gerard (Bynum 1985). As her body literally fell to pieces, those pieces themselves were said to smell sweet and could effect healing on others. A widow named Catherine had a vision that Lidwina's breasts would fill with milk on the evening of the nativity. After Lidwina received a vision, they did so, and Catherine drank of the milk and needed no other substance for days. She was also known for providing food and drink to the poor, and her charity was reported as pleasing to God. Towards the end of Lidwina's life, after a long illness, it was reported that the frequent administration of the Eucharist kept her alive. She gave food to others, and healed others through contact with her own bodily effluvia.

Another example is that of Catherine of Siena, mentioned previously. Hagiography of Catherine bears some similarities to the story of Lidwina. She was also known for fasting, devotion to the Eucharist, and for miracles associated with food. Catherine spoke of her own suffering, hunger, and yearning for Christ as akin to a hunger for food. The suffering she encountered was also framed as redemptive. In her writing, Catherine used images such as sucking milk from the breast of Christ to nourish the soul, making her more able to nourish others in return. She also described a desire for Christ like the thirst of a drunken man, which cannot be quenched (Bynum 1985, 8-9). Other saints have stories with similar themes, and this trope became common with stories of holy women. Bynum claims this fixation on food, suffering, and denial cannot simply be put down to medieval expressions of eating disorders, but rather to a more active means of engaging with religious belief and of asserting personal power or resistance to expectations.

Food was the one major material resource that women controlled:

> Women were associated with food preparation and distribution rather than food consumption ... Chronicle accounts of medieval banquets ... indicate that the sexes were often segregated and that women were sometimes relegated to watching from the balconies while gorgeous foods were rolled out to please the eyes as well as the palates of men. Indeed men were rather afraid of women's control of food. Canon lawyers suggested, in the codes they drew up, that a major danger posed by women was their manipulation of male virility by charms and potions added to food (Bynum 1985, 10).

While feeding others was expected behaviour, women feeding themselves was often considered less important. Taking the role to the extreme, Lidwina, for example, fed others both with food and with her own body, denying her own nourishment to gain spiritual power; to live the suffering of Christ to become closer to him, but also to exert control over the people around her in a religiously sanctioned way. This behaviour was not condoned by the Church, perhaps in part because it didn't want to encourage women to become the focus of religious attention, but also perhaps because of the danger involved in such extreme fasting. In the case of Catherine of Siena, she gathered much attention and a reputation for piety. It was believed she developed stigmata, and had regular visions of Christ. She also starved herself to death at the age of 33 (Espi-Forcen 2012).

Some women may have resorted to extreme fasting in the name of religion because of a fear of the body. The Church considered bodies a source of sin, something apart from the soul, which could lead one through its desires to the sin of excess. To distance oneself from sinfulness and temptation, denial of the body could be an attractive option, long extoled by ascetics and theologians. To deny the body while also becoming an agent of spiritual knowledge, local attention, and some authority, allowed these women to exercise more control over their families and their lives. It seems paradoxical to say that by denying the body women could become fully embodied actors in a social drama while also obtaining cultural capital, but this was the case. Was this done in a calculated manner? We shouldn't discount the strong religious feelings and beliefs of these women. Perhaps in some cases it was calculated behaviour; in others it may have been unconscious means to operate within a world that limited their options. If women were associated with, and criticized for, their deeper connection to body rather than intellect or spirit, a focus on food and the body then became a vehicle by which women could turn that body into spirit, into spiritual strength rather than embodied weakness.

Religion and medical recommendations for diet

Finally, back to the medical view of women and what they should eat. How much did religion affect or restrict their ability to follow medical regimes and recommended diets? Were the two influences equal? Were they often in conflict? It is far less likely that significant numbers of people followed medically prescribed diets. To begin with, only the elite had the means to get specific dietary recommendations by a physician. Would there have been a conflict between the Church calendar of fast days and feast days and medical recommendations for health? In most cases, probably not. Medieval cooking, at least if cookbooks were any indication, contained an extraordinary variety of ingredients and methods for preparing food that met fasting regulations. While, of course, wealthier individuals would have cooks to prepare these foods, as well as the means to purchase expensive ingredients, recommendations for pregnancy and postpartum eating and offsetting the cold and moist nature of women could be accommodated during fast days. In fact, anyone who could afford spices and sauces had the means to modify the humoral makeup of any given food, rendering it at least more suitable to consume.

Of more concern, then, is the association between food and the inherent sinfulness of women. Women, it seems, were placed in a bind. If following the teachings of the Church, fasting, spiritually beneficial for anyone, was one way to ameliorate or control the sexual nature of women. Theoretically, fasting and/or maintaining a largely vegetarian diet (such as diets eaten by both male and female monastics) was an aid not just in the keeping of the soul and growing spiritually through the imitation of Christ's suffering, but also in maintaining chastity. In avoiding those foods thought to enflame the passions[13], women and men would keep a greater check on their spirituality. One question arises: was this considered most important among both religious and wealthy women? According to the strict rules of comportment urged by the authors of the conduct literature covered in Chapter Seven, bourgeois wives should not shame their husbands by appearing bold, instead remaining self-contained and chaste. Would this emphasis on controlled and chaste behaviour have extended to stricter control of eating, not just of how much one ate, but also the food one chose? Would this have been in conflict with the desire to impress others by providing aspirational cuisine – mimics of the expensive and elaborate food of the aristocratic feast?

There is some evidence, at least in artwork, that townsmen and women who served others, or were purveyors of foodstuffs, were often portrayed as rather portly. Peasants as well usually lack the figures of aristocratic women, although some were portrayed as thin. They do, however, lack the refined beauty of the aristocrat. Is this more of a commentary on food consumption in the lower classes, or just the view of less refined bodies, and less refined individuals? We know that monks, at least in comic portrayals, are mocked for being fat, implying that the supposedly spare diet of monastic communities was often flouted. I am not arguing that today's association

13 Including, for some reason, leeks.

with thinness and control of diet in women of higher socioeconomic status was associated specifically with the aristocratic classes in the Middle Ages: the connection isn't that simple. But there is an association between class and diet, and between religion and diet. Those relationships also have gendered aspects, as this chapter argues. These relationships, along with comparisons to other cultures and that of the present day, are explored further in Chapter Nine.

9 Evolving Advice for Women's Health Through Diet

Abstract

This chapter is a summary overview of how dietary advice for women changed from Galen through the Early Modern period. Literature from both anthropology and folklore are used to compare how both contemporary and historical foodways can inform our understanding of medieval medicine, and how women face some of the same cultural obstacles today regarding pregnancy and health as they have in other eras. Looking at folk medicine and traditional foodways can help us better understanding many aspects of the life of subaltern classes in the Middle Ages and beyond, and how food, medicine, and diet are ultimately culture-bound, even when they purport to be scientific.

Keywords: folk medicine, gender roles, traditional Chinese medicine, Ayurveda, Latina folklore, traditional healers

How did medieval recommendations for women's diets fare in the Early Modern period and beyond? Since specific dietary advice for women, at least in gynaecological manuals, is often for the same kinds of food recommended for the ill or convalescing, there is some parallel to be found in later time periods. Dietary recommendations remained fairly stable, even though by 1650 the understanding of how the body processed food was changing. Sources written specifically for women as housewives and household managers began to appear more frequently in the latter half of the Early Modern era. We will see that, at least in those books, the association of women with care, nourishment, and healing is more explicit.

The waning of the longstanding humoral theory is explored in so far as it may have led to a different understanding of how women should eat. Mechanical theories of digestion, which posited that the stomach grinds up food rather than concocting it, applied to both men and women. Later

Vaughan, Theresa A., *Women, Food, and Diet in the Middle Ages: Balancing the Humours.* Taylor & Francis Group, 2020
DOI: 10.5117/9789462989382_CH09

theories, such as chemical and digestive (rather than concoction of food), would have likewise made little distinction between the digestive process of men and women, though of course there was some advice on what was good for women to eat. There was a longstanding belief that the digestion of aristocratic men and women was somehow more delicate and their palate more refined than those of the lower classes. It is important to keep in mind that, while theoretical and medical explanations for dietary ideas can and did change, general trends in diet and in judging appropriate foods for different age groups, different genders, and for the elite as opposed to the common person lagged well behind changing medical advice. The diet of the common person was also more conservative than the more fashionable diet of the elite. This is, perhaps, one indication that medical recommendations were treated then in much the same way as they are now. Some people, particularly people who can afford to do so, will consider medical recommendations and perhaps modify their diet accordingly, while the majority continue to eat as they always have, either unaware of medical recommendations or simply indifferent to them. Foodways do change over time, but those changes are only indirectly related to medical advances for most people. Instead, foodways change more readily as elite food culture's ingredients and dishes become copied by lower social strata during times of abundance, and the ingredients and dishes of lower social strata are gradually adopted by elites during times of scarcity (Wiegelmann 2015 [1974]).

Consciousness of obesity as a problem in and of itself would gradually become more prevalent, but that may be secondary to the changing demands of fashion: a thin waist, proper pallor, breast size, and the ability to fit into currently fashionable clothing could all affect dietary choices, as well as lead women to strive for other forms of body modification. This brief summary focuses on Western Europe and North America.

In the contemporary era, dietary advice for women during pregnancy is differentiated from advice for invalids. While 'gentle' foods are still recommended for women with nausea or heartburn, recommendations and restrictions on women's diets have multiplied considerably with both a focus on contagions and on a consciousness of substances that are dangerous and potentially teratogenic, as well as those nutrients, such as folic acid, that help prevent birth defects. I suggest that, while certainly informed by medical science to some degree, restrictions on what and how pregnant women should eat derives partially from tradition and folk medicine, combined with long-standing food fears of contamination, along with a sense that the first responsibility of pregnant women is to consume nothing with even the slightest chance of causing harm to a foetus. This is actually a very old idea, in the Western tradition going back to the Greeks[1] – that food can serve to both heal and hurt, and that you are what you eat. It also may be a new twist in our very child-centred contemporary culture.

If we look globally, some ideas about diet and women's health are cross-cultural, and some of course vary considerably. That women should make some modifications to the diet during pregnancy is common to many cultures, although theories on the best foods to consume vary. There are also examples of diets where food appropriate for women is different from that for men (Meyer-Rochow 2009). In many cultures, for example, men are allotted not only a greater quantity of food but also food of higher caloric density and higher protein[2]. We might wonder if the recommendations for more easily concocted and delicate food for women are based on an assumption (whether correct or incorrect) of their more delicate constitutions, or simply a way of preserving the higher quality food for men. It wouldn't be the first time that rules for women, overtly stated from consideration for their more delicate natures, were actually meant to impose restrictions keeping them in some way subservient. Perhaps not, but a brief cross-cultural comparison might suggest avenues for alternate interpretations and also for future research.

What lessons can we take away from this material in understanding contemporary dietary recommendations for women? Is the scientific foundation of current recommendations based on a wholly culturally neutral analysis of scientific data, or is it, at least in part, a culturally-based analysis in which old ideas about women and nutritional health are given new form? The entire understanding of the workings of the human body, nutrition, and digestion have changed irrevocably from Greco-Roman humoral theory, but how have diets and dietary recommendations remained stable? How have they changed? What elements of cultural understanding and assumptions are still implicit in our view of food as a source of both healing and of potential ill health? How have notions of gender, physiology, and diet changed, but how have they remained the same? And in what sense are women still associated with food, nurturance, and healing?

1 While the notions of food and medicine beginning with ancient Greek medicine had much influence on Western Europe, there are medical theories as old or older in other parts of the world that affected the foodways of other cultures. India and China are well-known examples, but folk theories of food to promote health are widespread.

2 In many cultures, including Western cultures, men tend to be more associated with meat than women. For interesting studies of this phenomenon in American culture, see Shapiro 2001 or Levenstein 2003.

Women's diet advice in the Early Modern Period

Despite the gradual abandonment of humoral theory as the basis for treatment of physical health through food, dietary advice did not change much during the Early Modern period. In fact, Ken Albala (2012) notes that while theoretical medicine changed considerably from the largely humour-based recommendations of the Middle Ages and the Early Modern period, to the mechanical, chemical, and digestive theories of later periods, food intended for the ill and convalescing remained largely the same, often with no particular theoretical basis, or a vague basis that simply changed as the foods stayed the same. Many of the dietary recommendations for women from the medieval period, as found in the gynaecological handbooks described previously, most closely mirror general advice for convalescents or those with a weakened ability to concoct their food, either because of a temperament favouring a cold, moist complexion (as was the norm for women), or a humoral imbalance resulting in the same condition. As discussed previously, humoral 'heat' was thought to be required to concoct one's food, concoction being the first stage of processing food into blood or other substances. The recommendations remained general, as no specific reference on diet for women was published during the Renaissance (Gentilcore 2015).

Albala makes a distinction between food recommendations for correcting specific humoral imbalances or acute conditions, and food recommendations for the convalescing. Those recommendations are based on the idea that some people have problems concocting their food, leading them to require food that is, in a sense, precooked. These problems may not be acute, but rather long-term conditions of digestion with little to no bearing on the otherwise normal physical strength or health of the patient. This is somewhat akin to the difference between, say, recommending a bland diet for someone with chronic heartburn or an ulcer, and 'feeding a cold and starving a fever', folk advice intended to address an acute condition through diet. In this sense, pregnancy was at the same time a normal condition, and one requiring a gentle but fortifying diet.

Convalescent diets of the Early Modern period can be gleaned in some part from cookbooks and from medical writing, including humanist works on the care of the human body, not always written by trained physicians. For example, Platina, mentioned in Chapter Six, wrote *De honesta voluptate*, essentially a treatise on improving health and caring for one's body, including a collection of recipes by Maestro Martino. Usually the recipes had little or nothing to do with theories of health, but were simply a collection by a contemporary that Platina saw fit to include because of the link he made between diet and health.

Like most early recipe collections, the recipes represented haute cuisine, cuisine meant for the aristocracy or the manor house to be prepared by a professional chef (such as Maestro Martino). In some cases, doctors would be consulted about individual diets, and a cook might receive instructions about what foods to serve or to avoid, but the recipe collections themselves may only include a section on recipes for invalids, without detail on the medical logic behind the preparation and serving of those dishes.

Recommendations included what were thought of as humorally neutral foods and foods that were proper for the very young or the very old. As was the case in the Middle Ages, these foods included broths, porridge and gruels, eggs, dairy products, and poultry if meat was included. As in the Middle Ages, what was considered appropriate food for the convalescing or invalid was generally white or light in colour – light bread, chicken, almonds. Perhaps not coincidentally, these were also foods for the wealthy, especially wealthy women (Laurioux 2011). Recommendations for lower class women were less specified by the written evidence, perhaps because peasant women were thought to have a hardier constitution better able to digest courser foods, but also because the entire written tradition was really only applicable to those who could read or afford physicians, hence the aristocracy and upper classes (Klemettilä 2012). Just as during the medieval period, finding evidence for folk traditions or traditional medicine in the Early Modern era applicable to the majority of people is a bit more difficult. While we can see some links between foods to avoid[3] in popular ideas about diet and health, specific recommendations are tougher to find. For many, simply having enough to eat, a desire expressed in the legend of Cockaigne (Lochrie 2016), may have been the primary focus for the lower classes, and perhaps for pregnant women in particular.

In the recipes for convalescent food from the sixteenth century, often what one finds is food that is simply a modification of conventional recipes. In the *Opera* of Bartolomeo Scappi (1500-1570, Dumenza, Italy), for example, there is an entire chapter on convalescent cooking[4], though the recipes

3 Some examples include avoiding strawberries to prevent birthmarks, or craving food one could not get, which might leave a mark on the body of the infant.

4 Book VI of the *Opera* is entitled *De convalescenti* (*Dishes for the Sick*). This book contains sections for prepared potions, concentrates (primarily meat broths), pastes (meat pastes), thick soups and stews, roasts, barley gruel, thick broths, pies, tourtes, sops (typically bread soaked in fruit syrup, broth, or other liquid), milk dishes, eggs, 'dainty pottages', fruits, sauces, jellies, and confections. While a variety of material is used, the ingredients run heavily to grain (barley, rice), poultry, fruit, almond milk (presumably for fast days), and sweet, palatable dishes. See Scappi 2011 [1570].

themselves do not specify the conditions addressed (Albala 2012, 325). Other cookbooks from the sixteenth century do give some medical explanations, such as those in *De vice Romanorum* by Alessandro Petronio (published 1572). In this book, there is some elaboration on the medical usage of various foods, somewhat akin to that found in the *Tacuina sanitatis,* but with the addition of recipes. Albala suggests that for many authors, such as Scappi, any food recommendations for convalescent cookery may have simply been derived from common sense and tradition more than any real understanding of humoral theory.

> They seem to be drawn from common sense intuition rather than theory. Of course, it may be that the original logic stemming from medical theory had barely been lost and through common use had become accepted generally, much as many home remedies and folk nostrums became embedded in the popular consciousness without understanding how they are supposed to work (2012, 325).

It also should be noted that those recipes found in cookbooks focus on medicinal foods – foods that nourish and strengthen the body – rather than on recipes for medicines, which were the province of physicians and apothecaries. In the medical literature of the Middle Ages explored earlier, recommendations for nutrition, while humorally based, were far outnumbered by instructions for the making of medicines, even if they included edible substances or used them to process ingredients. Wine, honey, vinegar, spices, and herbs were all common ingredients in those recipes, but were rarely part of more general dietary advice.

Cookbooks after 1650 exhibit some changes from those of the previous two centuries. Formal cookbooks, written by professional chefs for professional chefs, or copied and modified for the household of the haute bourgeoisie (such as we find in the *Ménagier de Paris*), often omitted cooking for convalescents altogether. In those rare instances where such recipes did appear, they seem to have remained unchanged from the earlier part of the Early Modern period, and indeed from the early recipe collections of the late Middle Ages. In England, however, cookbooks began to be written for women who directed households, by definition not the grand cookery of the court or the manor house, but instead for the literate woman of lesser means, probably a reasonably well-to-do townswoman, for example. *The English Huswife: containing the inward and outward vertues which ought to be in a compleat woman* was written by Gervaise Markham (c. 1568-1637, Nottinghamshire) and first published in 1615. It includes medicine for treatment of some diseases (1986 [1615]). Another such book, Eliza Smith's (d. c. 1732) *The Compleat Housewife* (1727), mixes household advice with recipes, convalescent cookery and home remedies, medicine for specific illnesses, and confectionary. Originally published in London, it became the first cookbook to be printed in the American colonies. The recipes themselves contain some continuity with the past. For example, there are various recipes for caudle, a drink or gruel made of, in this case, oatmeal, nutmeg, and sugar. Caudle, while its constituent ingredients did change somewhat over time, had its antecedents in the medieval period. Caudle has some significance because of its association with women and childbirth (Martin 2009).

The death of humoral theory

Humoral theory was gradually displaced in the Modern era, especially as new understandings of the functioning of the body came to light during the Scientific Revolution. A new understanding of disease, contagion theory, gradually displaced humoral theory. Eventually the humours were discounted as an accurate description of the functioning of the body, though certain medical practices based on humoral theory, such as blood-letting or cupping, were commonly used through the nineteenth century. Some of those same theories exist in various forms even in the present day. The increasing number of dissections beginning in the 1600s, along with increasingly sophisticated instruments, such as the microscope, led to changes in understanding the composition and function of the body. Likewise, two different theories of how the body processed food, mechanical and chemical, gradually displaced the concoction of humoral theory (Clericuzio 2012).

The first marked change in digestive theory can be traced back to Paracelsus, influenced by the work of Marcilio Ficino (1433-1499, Republic of Florence). Discussing the non-naturals, Ficino stated that food was rich in spirit and oily substances. Paracelsus, rather than accepting that digestion took place through concoction, or heat, posited that pure and impure matter were separated by an 'internal alchemist' able to separate poison from spirit. Jean-Baptiste von Helmont (1578-1644, Brussels) later suggested that chemical reactions prompted by stomach acid led to the release of vital spirit, the source of life.

Mechanical digestion, traced back to the influence of René Descartes (1596-1650, La Hayne en Touraine, France), viewed the process of digestion as a result of the grinding action of the stomach. In the digestive system, food was matter in motion, subject to change. By the mid-seventeenth century, physicians saw digestion as both a mechanical and chemical process. Further refinement of these theories, for example, the iatrochemists' focus on acids versus alkalis in the body, would continue through the end of the seventeenth century and beyond (Clericuzio 2012).

These changes in understanding digestion were accompanied by speculation on the nature of the disease process. Jean Fernel, for example, came to believe that humoralism, which explained disease as resulting from an imbalance of the humours, could not account for most diseases. However, contagion theory, or the theory that disease was caused by contact with illness, didn't really gain traction until the nineteenth century. Although elements of contagion theory can be found going all the way back to Avicenna, Galen's theories proved hard to reject. In the Early Modern period, as a result of the increasing practice of dissection of human bodies, Galen's teachings on anatomy began to be challenged. For example, *De humani corpus fabrica*, written by Andreas Vesalius (1514-1564, Hapsburg, Netherlands) and published in 1543, presented a description of the human body based upon systematic dissection (Gaynes 2011). A weakening attachment to Galen allowed different digestive theories and contagion theory to eventually become dominant.

Consciousness of health, consciousness of fashion

The relationship between diet and standards of beauty, explored in Chapter Seven, was only a fraction of a much longer story about restrictions and imperatives placed on women and their bodies to conform to ever-changing beauty standards. Women, like men, experience their bodies in the context of the social standards required to present them. We are ingrained with *habitus* from a young age: how to comport ourselves, what we should look like, what bodies are acceptable and unacceptable within social and cultural norms. Standards of beauty today are often couched within the language of health – an attractive body is a fit body, in which eating is controlled and the body is exercised. There are myriad books to tell us how we should eat, whether it be like our supposed caveman ancestors, by cutting out fat, by eschewing too many processed carbohydrates, by fasting intermittently (this time for health rather than penance – although there is more in common between the two than meets the eye), by drinking juice or avoiding liquid calories, and by giving up alcohol or drinking enough of it to make our hearts healthy. While the specifics of beauty standards change, most of them for women in the last one hundred years have focused on thinness. That thinness may be a small waist but larger hips and breasts, or having the flat, lean look of an adolescent boy, but some form of thinness has been the dominant norm in much of Western Europe and Anglo-American[5] cultures.

Even our skin, a dominant feature of beauty in the conduct literature of the Middle Ages and in much of medieval discourse on beauty, should be tanned in imitation of those with enough wealth for lives of leisure, as opposed to the once desired paleness of those wealthy enough not to engage in outdoor manual labour. Our skin should, however, like the standards of the Middle Ages, be youthful in appearance, and there is a vast industry in the West selling concoctions and cosmetics designed to keep that skin soft, blemish-free, and without wrinkles. Diet is also implicated in contemporary standards of beauty beyond simply making our figures conform to a certain size, or our weight within a range that medical science deems healthy. The proper diet, we are told, will make us look and feel younger. Proper nutrition makes our skin glow, avoiding sugar or fat clears blemishes and hydrates our skin. Diet and morality are intertwined, although this time in a way less overtly religious.

According to Peter Stearns:

> People could indulge their taste for fashion and other products with a realization that, if they disciplined their bodies through an attack on fat, they could preserve or even enhance their health and also establish their moral credentials ... An appropriately slender figure could denote the kind of firm character, capable of self-control, that one would seek in a good worker in an age of growing indulgence; ready employability and weight management could be conflated (2002, 59-60).

The media (and social talk) tends to portray fat people in general, and women in particular, as engaging in immoral behaviour, of not having enough self-control to eat properly, and in accordance with social standards:

> Moreover, while heaping the blame on individuals, news reports also draw upon and reproduce stereotypes of fat people as gluttonous, slothful, and ignorant, and of parents of fat children as neglectful and irresponsible. Thus, such reports reproduce the negative moral valence of fatness (Saguy and Gruys 2010).

Despite the social pressure to be thin, to eat right, and the social censure that goes along with obesity or poor diet, people still are apt to eat the way

5 By Anglo-America, I am referring to the English-speaking cultures in the United States and Canada stemming from the colonial period.

they want to eat. Although the sins are the same – sloth, gluttony – they are, at least in the United States, associated less with being sinful in the religious sense, and more with sinning against the social order. Obese people, we are told, cost far more money than people who can keep their eating under control. If they have health insurance, they drive up the costs through the comorbidity of obesity and its complications: diabetes, heart disease, cancer, and hypertension. Why should we pay for other people's lifestyle choices, we are asked? In the United States, if they don't have health insurance, they still drive up the cost for the average taxpayer either by being lazy and reliant upon welfare, disability, or Medicaid, or simply by demanding emergency care when their illnesses become life-threatening. It is the unpaid medical bills associated with these people, who are also no doubt lazy because they are poor, that cost the rest of us. While this is the reality of health care in the United States, countries with socialized medicine frame the public health arguments in similar ways[6]. Witness the debate over how much obesity costs the National Health Service each year in Great Britain, or the same debate in Canada over the network of health care often referred to as 'Medicare'.

I have not touched upon race as it pertains to gender, obesity, and beauty standards, but again – at least in the United States – to have a brown or black female body is to be suspect. When that brown or black female body also does not conform to social standards of beauty, or medical standards of healthy size, that body is doubly suspect. After all, goes the stereotype, brown bodies are more apt to be a drain on social resources through laziness (and therefore poverty), higher birth rate (and lack of sexual self-control), and by having more of a tendency to be fat (gluttony) (Goodman, Johnston, and Cairns 2017). While medieval medical manuals, diets, and standards of beauty are not couched in these terms, they certainly are today. The situation is somewhat different in Western Europe, in part because of differences in the cost and delivery of health care, which is managed by the state, but the same beauty standards, and the same conflict between obesity and beauty still exists.

Pregnancy and diet in the modern era

As medieval dietary recommendations for women during the Middle Ages usually focused on pregnancy, it is instructive to view later recommendations for pregnancy and diet in the contemporary West. Practices certainly vary

6 See, for example, Scarborough et al. 2011.

across the cultures of Western Europe and North America, though there are certain common features. Diet during pregnancy was as much a concern in the Middle Ages as it is today. Also of concern throughout the twentieth and early twenty-first centuries is the amount of weight gained during pregnancy. In the United States, women of a healthy weight when they begin pregnancy are told to gain no more than thirty pounds[7]. This takes into account the weight of the baby, enlarged uterus, placenta, amniotic fluid, water retention, and some extra fat in preparation for lactation. Anything beyond that, women are told, is simply fat. The stricture to stay thin essentially carries over into pregnancy: a healthy, self-disciplined woman will not 'let herself go' during pregnancy, or use pregnancy as an excuse to eat whatever she may like, meaning consuming foods that society and medical science consider unhealthy. This contrasts simultaneously with the folk wisdom of giving a pregnant woman what she wants to eat, lest her cravings imprint themselves upon the foetus. After pregnancy, women are encouraged to restrict eating to lose the 'baby weight' as quickly as possible. The rules of eating remain the same, and control over one's diet is a moral imperative, traces of the religious stance against gluttony by medieval clerics!

Women are also, while pregnant, restricted in terms of the types of food they eat. There was a general sense that one should eat easily digested foods during pregnancy, and avoid foods that might harm the child through sympathetic magic. Today, the fear over ingesting harmful substances has been reframed in terms of contamination and contagion. Pregnancy itself has become focused not so much upon the health of the mother as that of the child, at least in societies where food is abundant. Even forty years ago, women in the West were advised not to drink or smoke excessively, and to perhaps avoid a few foods, such as undercooked pork, which might cause illness. The pregnant body was controlled more through its size than in the specific foods and other substances that passed into its body. Today, pregnant women are often given a list of foods they cannot eat. These include raw or undercooked meat (food-borne illnesses like Toxoplasma, Salmonella or E. coli), shellfish (various contamination issues), tuna (mercury content), deli meats (Listeria), too much sugar or sweet foods (gestational diabetes), alcohol (in the U.S., no amount is considered safe so women are told to

7 The recommendations for weight gain were based upon those first published in the United States in 1990 by the Institutes of Medicine. Subsequently, new guidelines were issued in 2009, and while thirty pounds is the midpoint for weight gain for women whose BMI falls in the normal range, the newer recommendations address a wide range of starting weights, adjusting recommended weight gains for each (Rasmussen and Yaktine 2009, 2).

totally abstain to avoid the possibility of foetal alcohol syndrome; in Europe one is advised to only drink moderately), raw fish (Salmonella, Listeria), organ meats (possible vitamin A toxicity), caffeine (in cola, coffee, or tea, it potentially restricts foetal growth), raw sprouts (Salmonella), unpasteurized milk, milk products, or juice (Salmonella), unwashed produce, (various food-borne illnesses caused by Listeria, Salmonella, or E. coli), junk food (generally unhealthy), and raw eggs or any foods containing raw eggs (FDA 2018). There is certainly a medical basis for these recommendations, but how much of it is also designed for social control over the female body, and enshrinement of the child?

Regulation of maternal weight, mentioned above, along with increasingly restrictive eating rules that treat female bodies as merely vessels for ideal gestation, both have implications for the control of female bodies:

> Core assumptions at the heart of obesity science regarding the scale of the obesity problem, the nature of the risk and where responsibility for health should fall, have been taken up uncritically in medical arenas focused on conception, pregnancy and reproduction. This in turn is providing new and disturbing opportunities for the surveillance, regulation and disciplining of 'threatening' (fat) female bodies while at the same time perpetuating a number of taken-for-granted medico-moral assumptions about individuals and the causes of fatness (McNaughton 2011, 164).

Dietary guidelines for women, whether derived from folk medicine or professional medicine, whether from the Middle Ages or more recent times, have multiple aims and meanings. On the surface, they speak to the role of food in women's health. Sometimes those guidelines are expressed in positive terms, such as recommendations for certain foods to make you healthy, but many are expressed in more negative terms: avoid eating too much/too little/the wrong kinds of food or risk fatness/illness/damage to a foetus. These rules are also culture-dependent, and vary by location, time period, and whatever medical system is in vogue. This is not to say, for example, that knowing the risks and benefits of certain food during pregnancy or otherwise can't be useful, nor that women routinely try to harm a foetus through consumption of specific food or drink, but managing degrees of risk through control of the body is at issue here.

Pregnancy and birth are uncertain times. Dietary recommendations during pregnancy, from whatever source and time period, are an effort to control risk and maximize the possibility of a healthy outcome. This is true in both folk and professional medicine. But in the process, women can become mere vessels, obligated to serve as perfect incubators for new life. For example, the average annual incidence of Listeriosis[8] among pregnant women in the United States from 2009-2011 was three per 100,000 people, higher than the average rate among the general population of .29 per 100,000 people. However, this still represents an exceedingly rare possibility of contracting Listeria when pregnant. Of these cases, most were contracted by eating soft cheeses. While the effects of Listeriosis on a foetus can be devastating, this only affected 227 pregnant women in the United States over the three-year period from 2009-2011, out of approximately four million pregnancies each year (CDC). Still, dietary guidelines for pregnant women in the United States involve eliminating all soft cheeses, unpasteurized milk products, deli meats, raw hot dogs, and other food items that may theoretically harbour Listeria bacteria. The risks are very small, but the recommendation is applied across a large population. At what point are such guidelines reasonable, and at what point do they become about social control of the pregnant body?

As many have noted, the body is both a physical object and a locus of symbolic meaning and action. Even though medical understanding has changed over time, we can't assume that science itself is independent of social and cultural context (Strathern 1996, 148). While modern biomedicine has to a certain degree separated medicine from food, in contrast with humoral medicine, food recommendations reflect a current understanding of diet and nutrition, but always seen through the lens of cultural imperatives placed on the body. Folk medicine, too, while having conservative elements, also reflects the concerns and expectations of the community. In the Middle Ages, with its emphasis on the beauty of the skin, a birthmark could mar otherwise clear skin, hence the proscriptions against eating strawberries, or the avoidance of unfulfilled cravings. The fact that folk medicine still exists is evidence that it is a living tradition still meeting cultural or community needs (Kingston 2017). Women, in what they eat, are constrained by both professional and folk medicine, and at least during reproductive years, are seen as potential receptacles of male sperm and of foetuses.

Are women's diets consistent across cultures?

The study of foodways in global cultures is a feature of interdisciplinary food studies, including work in the fields of anthropology and folklore. Nutritional

8 An infection caused by contact with the Listeria monocytogenes bacterium. Listeriosis can cause death of a fetus or an overwhelming infection shortly after birth.

anthropology, for example, looks at the nuts and bolts of food availability and diet as it impacts gender and age differences, with an emphasis on developing societies, immigrant communities, and the Global South:

> As anthropologists, we are predominantly interested in how biology and culture intersect. ... On a more theoretical level, we can say that culture blends into biology. ... What is culturally defined as food and what is eaten may have reverberations in domains as diverse as ethnic identity, growth, and health (Dufour, Goodman, and Pelto 2013, vii).

For much of human history, of course, the ability to obtain sufficient food has been a concern of the majority of people. While the elite in any culture have had access to food (or, indeed, in more egalitarian cultures, higher status men have had better access to food), the majority of people have lived at or near the subsistence level. In such an environment, as was the case for most people during the Middle Ages, a sufficiency of food came before any notion of dietary theory, if in fact dietary theory was even known to the general population. Certain foods in the Middle Ages were considered higher status, a fact discussed at various points in this book, and for the most part they have high quality protein sources or fat sources such as meat. Vegetables and cereal grains have formed the better part of the diet in agricultural societies everywhere, and such was the case in the Middle Ages.

In looking at global diets and gender, there are many ways of differentiating what constitutes appropriate food by gender. Whether the emphasis is on food forbidden to women, either considered unhealthy or otherwise forbidden for fear it would injure women, or it was reserved for men, there are differing ways in which people think about food and gender. Food is 'good to think', in the sense that an analysis of foodways tells us important things about the culture. Lévi-Strauss famously looked at the contrast between the 'raw and the cooked' in a number of cultures as a vehicle for understanding binaries such as nature/culture (1983 [1969]). While Levi-Strauss' structuralism has long been critiqued, it is merely one example of the ways food serves as a nexus to understand agency, power relations, gender relations, and symbolic value.

If we confine ourselves to just a few examples pertaining specifically to women and diet, a variety of studies exist at the intersection of folklore, anthropology, and biomedicine. As the role of diet in pregnancy, childbirth, and post-partum was the focus of the medieval works cited above, the examples provided here focus on the same topics.

If we look at indigenous and Latina cultures in the state of New Mexico, the lore of lay midwives contains examples of special foods intended to enhance recovery and milk production during the post-partum period. For example, women in the 1960s were advised to eat corn gruels, brown sugar, and bread to enhance milk production. All of these foods were readily available, and in fact corn and bread were staples of New Mexico cultures. In addition, women were advised to consume meats from male animals to enhance their recovery (Marquez and Pacheco 1964). In a similar example, Chinese women were traditionally confined to the home and rest for the first month after childbirth. Ideally, they would spend much of that month in bed, eating a 'hot' diet to remedy the imbalance caused by bearing a child. While the Chinese system of hot and cold foods, of balance between yin and yang, was not identical to that of the ancient Greek system, there are some similarities. Foods are classified as warming, cooling, or neutral. A balanced body promoted the proper flow of Qi. Hot foods[9], associated with yin and male energy, were a way to address an imbalance caused by childbirth (Pillsbury 1978). In an example from Taiwan, the Chinese system of diet and health influences most food choices for women, not just those surrounding pregnancy and childbirth (Li et al. 2017).

In an example involving not so much food choice as food restriction, in South India, it was common practice among poor women to restrict food consumption during pregnancy. This was not done as a response to food scarcity, but in an effort to produce smaller, more easily birthed children. In areas where access to medical care was very limited, having low birthweight babies was seen as a means to avoid birth complications (Nichter and Nichter 1983). In other parts of Asia, certain foods, like papaya, are believed to be unsafe to consume during pregnancy (Adebiyi, Adaikan, and Prasad 2002). In fact, people in almost all cultures have beliefs about what foods to consume and avoid during pregnancy and while nursing. Some of these beliefs have a scientific basis, but many more, including those among Western cultures, have a basis in folk belief (Monti 2000).

A variety of material is available in Western medical journals that spans cultures, some of which seriously considers traditional forms of diet as medicine, and traditional medicine itself. Much of it, however, seeks to remedy what are seen in Western medicine as chronic deficiencies in diet. These deficiencies can take two forms: first, deficiency in calories or nutrition in a traditional diet, or actual deficiency in nutrients or imbalance in calories derived from adopting a Western diet. Vitamin deficiencies in the developing world, for example, are the subject of efforts to improve

9 Hot and cold foods, in the Chinese system, are not necessarily associated with the temperature of the food itself, but rather their innate properties that heated or cooled the body.

dietary quality through genetically modified rice that includes Vitamin A to counteract vision problems. Western farming practices and irrigation have increased crop yields. Some of this influence is based on making sure people get enough calories, and then that they receive adequate nutrition. While this may be a laudable goal, cultural misunderstandings can cloud relationships between the people being helped and those helping.

Changing or destabilizing traditional food systems can destabilize a community both in terms of power and in farming or processing cooking practices. It also may make low-income farmers reliant on purchasing seed, rather than saving back part of the harvest. Traditional farming methods, which tend to be best suited to local climate and soil conditions, may be lost or ignored. This leads us to the second deficiency of diet, which has become increasingly common: the adoption of a Western diet not in terms of meeting nutritional baselines, but in increasing consumption of foods that may lead to diabetes, obesity, heart disease, and other ills of Western society, though the United States is generally blamed as the primary culprit. Ultimately, these are detrimental to health. Some critiques aim at the actual producers and marketers of these foods – Coca-Cola, McDonalds, and so forth (Leatherman and Goodman 2013 [2005]). Other studies blame an American diet and its influences (Gladwell 2013 [1998]). Another example is changes in infant feeding practices, with formula companies touting the scientific healthfulness of their product, which leads women to decrease or stop breastfeeding in favour of the more 'scientific' diet; this tends to be expensive, so mothers may over-dilute the formula or prepare it with contaminated water (Halpern 1982).

When women, who are the food providers and nurturers for their families worldwide, adopt changing diets, those changes may have a problematic effect on health, especially with the adoption of a standard American diet. Devaluing traditional remedies and food practices, as well as traditional medicine and treatments for disease or conditions such as pregnancies, can lead to changing roles for women and decreased health. In a non-Western example, Australian Aboriginal diets have changed radically, as they adopt the Western diet of highly refined and processed foods, especially as these are relatively inexpensive to purchase or prepare. Traditional methods of food preparation and procurement are abandoned, to the detriment of health. In a famous experiment, a group of Aboriginal people were taken to the outback to live traditionally, where their health dramatically improved over a short period of time. Endemic conditions like Type 2 diabetes improved or disappeared altogether (O'Dea 1984). Not all traditional diets and traditional medicine have been good for women. In a number of places in Africa, the

Middle East, and Asia, women were expected to leave the high-quality food to the men, restricting calories available to them and potentially leading to disease (UNFAO 2013).

In most places, however, if we look at the diet intended for those who are ill or recuperating, including the diets of pregnant women, we see parallels with the Middle Ages – pregnancy is considered a somewhat weakened state, so women are encouraged to eat gentle but fortifying foods during pregnancy or the postpartum period. In the West today, this takes the form of avoiding those foods that may potentially be detrimental, but symbolically women crave odd foods or combinations of foods during pregnancy. Staple foods or foods consumed as young children are considered comforting, the exception being drinking plain milk, as most people in the world cannot digest it. Some cultures prepare special soups or broths considered to be especially good for pregnant or postpartum women; in rural Indian culture, for example, 83% of pregnant women and new mothers report eating special foods thought to be good for pregnant women. Most cultures have these foods. It was also common practice, however, for pregnant women to restrict their eating because they thought it would make for a smaller child and easier birth. While this was likely true, it also meant a less positive outcome in terms of both maternal and infant health (Mukhopadhyay and Sarkar 2009).

Conclusion

Women today, just like women in the Middle Ages, are subject to the various imperatives of culture. Dietary recommendations from the medical community influence what women eat or don't eat, during pregnancy or at any other time. Those recommendations may be informed by science but also by general cultural assumptions of what a female body should look like. We all live in a world where we must balance medical recommendations against cultural foodways, folk ideas about health and medicine, and pressure to maintain a socially-acceptable body.

Looking at dietary recommendations for women in the Middle Ages, we can clearly see that medical theories of diet and health have changed considerably, though the existence of a link between diet and health seems to be found in the majority of cultures and time periods. How that link is understood may vary, but the idea that there must be a relationship is, if not universal, then nearly so. Humoral theory bears resemblance, therefore, to some of the most elaborated systems of diet and health in the world, such as those of ancient China or India. It also bears resemblance to folk ideas of health and medicine in many cultures (Brady 2001).

Just as religion also had a significant role in the timing of what one could consume in the medieval period, as well as in the prohibition against gluttony, so efforts to control body size today can take on an almost religious quality. While obesity was somewhat less of a concern in the Middle Ages, the religious language of sin and redemption, of self-mastery and resistance to evil, seems to have transferred to the social imperative of thinness:

> Ultimately, women's attempts to lose weight by restricting their eating can generate a sense of agency, giving them the power of self-definition, but they do so by reproducing an all-too-familiar scenario, in which a woman's 'salvation' depends on her sacrifice and submission. In this sense, the Religion of Thinness resurrects and embodies the ghost of patriarchal religion, wherein a woman's creativity must be tied to her suffering, her power exercised through obedience, her redemption achieved through self-annihilation (Lelwica 2006).

Using the language of agency, we know that medieval women, just as women today, had choices to make about their lives. Dietary choices were one such expression of agency. As we have seen, it is far easier to document dietary guidelines set down by literature culture – within medicine or religion – than to determine what guidelines women actually followed in their everyday lives. This is especially challenging for women of the lower classes, or members of non-literate traditions. We probably know the most about individual agency in food choices by looking at the lives of women who claimed 'holy anorexia', but that is not the focus of this book.

By concentrating on the specific dietary advice in medieval works addressing health, and particularly women's health, we are afforded a window onto how food was used within the system of humoral medicine. As many of the recommendations covered in this book relate specifically to gynaecological and obstetric health, we can conclude that women and men's diets were probably not considered separately except during conditions such as pregnancy, that only affected women. However, by taking a view informed by anthropology and folklore, it is possible to set these recommendations into a cultural context, informed and influenced by local dietary patterns, religion, and folk medicine. While evidence for these areas is not abundant, it is possible to make some educated guesses.

In addition, one cannot examine diet without accounting for the role of the female body within the larger culture, and of women as associated with providing food and basic health care for non-aristocratic families. We must also consider societal expectations of the appearance of female bodies, both set within the religious imperatives of the time period, and the aesthetics of womanhood. These concerns are also related in some way to diet.

To return to the original question, 'What can we know about women and food in the Middle Ages'?, the answer is quite a bit, though not as much as we would like. We know most women were involved in the production of food, especially among peasants and the emerging middle class in cities and towns. They helped to sow and harvest, kept kitchen gardens and tended animals such as chickens and cows for domestic use, both for eggs in the former instance, and milk for cheese in the latter. We know that for most of the population, women were the primary food preparers, responsible for daily cooking and the feeding and nurturing of young children. For the upper classes, women were typically charged with supervising cooks and choosing menus. Most women were intimately involved in provisioning and preparing food for the household, or supervised others charged with those tasks.

We also have reasonable evidence, through the written record, illuminations, and folklore that women were also the primary practitioners of informal and traditional or folk medicine. They served as midwives, as holders of folk medical traditions in which they made simple diagnoses and prepared household remedies, sometimes for their own families, and sometimes for others in their communities. They may have been largely excluded from academic medicine, but were commonly involved in routine births and treatment of common illnesses. There is even some evidence, as we have seen with Hildegard of Bingen or the author(s) of the *Trotula*, that the line between academic medicine and folk medicine was permeable, and even literate medical practitioners may have drawn from the folk tradition.

Theoretical medicine, based in this period on Greek foundations of the humoral system, treated pregnancy as a state of infirmity, and saw the menstrual cycle as essential to women's health. We know that the use of diet was promoted for both women and men to address humoral imbalances that might lead to disease, and that food recommendations were sometimes different for women based upon assumptions about their humoral make-up and functioning of their reproductive system. A proper diet (according to the medical theories of the day) could treat absent or too abundant menstrual flow, could reduce bleeding after childbirth, and could help address infertility from a number of causes, from obesity to unhealthy thinness. We have also seen that food was not the only treatment for disease and disorder: medicines based on herbs or other substances were also very common.

Food regularly appears in folk beliefs about women and health, both in the Middle Ages and today. Folk medicine advises ways to deal with cravings during pregnancy, and the consequences of those cravings should they go unfulfilled. Food can serve as an aphrodisiac or as a deterrent to sexual desire. Visions of abundance show up in the folklore of the time, as an aspirational place for people struggling to get enough to eat, or as a means for the upper classes to poke fun at the lower classes.

An understanding of women, diet, and health cannot be separated from cultural expectations of women's bodies, both fed and abstinent. Women were expected to be neither too thin nor too fat, to comport themselves well, have a rosy glow associated with health, and to conform to social expectations of propriety, at least for the bourgeoisie and aristocracy. Women and men are both affected by social standards of beauty, and ideas about what a healthy person looks like.

The relationship between women, food, and health has always been complex. Women's bodies can be viewed as symbolic centres of agency, identity, and gender relations. Insofar as it is possible to understand these interrelationships, the Middle Ages provide a picture that, though vastly different in medical understanding, still maintains parallels with other cultures and other time periods. To understand the many variables surrounding food and diet is to understand something fundamental about gender, belief, and embodiment.

Bibliography

Adamson, Melitta Weiss. 1995. *Medieval Dietetics: Food and Drink in Regimen Sanitatis Literature from 800-1400*. Frankfurt Am Main: Peter Lang.

Adebiyi, Adebowale, P. Ganesan Adaikan, and R.N.V. Prasad. 2002. 'Papaya (*Carica papaya*) consumption is unsafe in pregnancy: fact or fable? Scientific evaluation of a common belief in some parts of Asia using a rat model'. *British Journal of Nutrition* 88: 199-203.

Albala, Ken. 2012. 'Food for healing: Convalescent cookery in the early modern era'. *Studies in History and Philosophy of Biological and Biomedical Sciences* 43: 323-328.

Albala, Ken, ed. 2014. *The Food History Reader: Primary Sources*. New York: Bloomsbury Academic.

Androniki, Dialeti. 2011. 'Defending Women, Negotiating Masculinity in Early Modern Italy'. *The Historical Journal* 54 (1): 1-23.

Arano, Luisa Cogliati. 1976. *The Medieval Health Handbook: Tacuinum Sanitatis*. Translated by Oscar Ratti and Adele Westbrook. New York: George Brazillen, Inc.

Åström, Berit. 2015. '"Sucking the Corrupte Mylke of an Infected Nurse": regulating the dangerous maternal body'. *Journal of Gender Studies* 24 (5): 574-586.

Avakian, Arlene Voski, and Barbara Haber, eds. 2005. *From Betty Crocker to Feminist Food Studies: Critical Perspectives on Women and Food*. Amherst: University of Massachussets Press.

Barkai, Ron. 1988. 'A Medieval Hebrew Treatise on Obstetrics'. *Medical History* 33: 96-119.

Bavaye-Kouidrat. 2016. 'Quelques aspects de la périnatalité à la cour de Bourgogne (1371-1482)'. In *Naissance et petite enfance à la cour de France: Moyen Âge-XIXe siècle*, edited by Pascale Mormiche and Stanis Perez, 25-34. Villeneuve d'Ascq, France: Septentrion.

Bell, Rudolph M. 1985. *Holy Anorexia*. Chicago: University of Chicago Press.

Benedek, Thomas G. 1978. 'Beliefs About Human Sexual Function in the Middle Ages and Renaissance'. In *Human Sexuality in the Middle Ages and Renaissance*, edited by Douglas Umstead, 97-116. Pittsburgh: Center for Medieval and Renaissance Studies, University of Pittsburgh.

Bennett, Bradley C. 2007. 'Doctrine of Signatures: An Explanation of Medicinal Plant Discovery or Dissemination of Knowledge?' *Economic Botony* 61 (3): 246-255.

Bennett, Judith. 1996. *Ale, Beer and Brewsters in England: Women's Work in a Changing World 1300-1600*. New York: Oxford University Press.

Berger, Margret. 1999. 'Introduction'. In *On Natural Philosophy and Medicine: Selections from the Causae et cure*, edited by Margret Berger, 1-18. Cambridge, UK: D.S. Brewer.

Berthiaud, Emmanuelle. 2016. "La grossesse invisible : la représentation des reines et des princesses enceintes à la cour de France (XVIIe-XIXe siècles)." In *Naissance et petite enfance à la cour de France: Moyen Age-XIXe siècle*, edited by Pascale Mormiche and Stanis Perez, 139-152. Villeneuve d'Ascq, France: Septentrion.

Biebel, Elizabeth M. 1998. 'Pilgrims to Table: Food Consumption in Chaucer's *Canterbury Tales*'. In *Food and Eating in Medieval Europe*, edited by Martha Carlin and Joel T. Rosenthal, 15-26. London: The Hambledon Press.

Bifulco, Maurizio, Magda Marasco, and Simona Pisanti. 2008. 'Dietary Recommendations in the Medieval Medical School of Salerno'. *American Journal of Preventative Medicine* 35 (6): 602-603.

Bingen, Hildegard of. 1998. *Hildegard von Bingen's Physica: The Complete English Translation of Her Classic Work on Health and Healing*. Translated by Priscilla Throop. Rochester, VT: Healing Arts Press.

Bingen, Hildegard of. 1999. *On Natural Philosophy and Medicine: Selections from the Cause et cure*. Translated by Margret Berger. Cambridge, UK: D.S. Brewer.

Bingen, Hildegard of. 2006. *Causes and Cures: The Complete English Translation of Hildegardis Causae et Curae Libri VI*. Translated by Priscilla Throop. Charlotte, VT: Medieval MS.

Bos, Gerrit. 1993. 'Ibn al-Jazzār on Women's Diseases and their Treatment'. *Medical History* 37: 296-312.

Brady, Erika, ed. 2001. *Healing Logics: Culture and Medicine in Modern Health Belief Systems*. Logan, UT: Utah State University Press.

Bylebyl, Jerome J. 1990. 'The Medical Meaning of Physica'. *Osiris* 6 (Renaissance Medical Learning: Evolution of a Tradition): 16-41.

Bynum, Carol Walker. 1985. 'Fast, Feast, and Flesh: The Religious Significance of Food to Medieval Women'. *Representations* 11 (Summer): 1-25.

Bynum, Carol Walker. 1987. *Holy Feast and Holy Fast: The Religious Significance of Food to Medieval Women*. Berkeley: University of California Press.

Caballero-Navas, Carmen. 2008. 'Medicine and Pharmacy for Women. The Encounter of Jewish Thinking and Practices with the Arabic and Christian Medical Traditions'. *European Review* 16 (2): 249-259.

Cabanillas, Isabel de la Cruz. 2017. 'Genre and text-type conventions in Early Modern Women's recipe books'. *Revista de Lingüística y Lenguas Aplicadas* 12: 13-21.

Cabré, Montserrat. 2000. 'From a Master to a Laywoman: A Feminine Manual of Self-Help'. *DYNAMIS: Acta Hispanica ad Medicinae Scientiarumque Historiam Illustrandam* 20: 371-395.

Cabré, Montserrat. 2008. 'Women or Healers? Household Practices and the Categories of Health Care in Late Medieval Iberia'. *Bulletin of the History of Medicine* 82 (1): 18-51.

Cadden, Joan. 1984. 'It Takes All Kinds: Sexuality and Gender Differences in Hildegard of Bingen's "Book of Compound Medicine"'. *Traditio* 40: 149-174.

Cairns, Kate, and Josée Johnston. 2015. *Food and Femininity*. New York: Bloomsbury Academic.

Canadé-Sautman, Francesca. 1992. 'Folklore and Medieval Medicine: Sources and Problems'. *Medieval Folklore* II: 91-102.

Carlin, Martha, and Joel T. Rosenthal, eds. 1998. *Food and Eating in Medieval Europe*. London: The Hambledon Press.

Carter, Susan. A. 2001. 'Willing Shape-shifters: The Loathly Lady from Irish Sovranty to Spenser's Duessa'. Ph.D., University of Toronto (304761550).

Cavallo, P., M. Proto, C. Patruno, & Maurizio Bifulco. 2008. 'The First Cosmetic Treatise of History. A Female Point of View'. *International Journal of Cosmetic Science* 30: 79-86.

CDC. 'Vital Signs: Listeria Illnesses, Deaths, and Outbreaks – United States, 2009-2011'. Centers for Disease Control and Prevention, accessed 10 February 2019. https://www.cdc.gov/mmwr/preview/mmwrhtml/mm6222a4.htm#tab1.

Chatten, Nicola. 2002. 'Fabliau'. In *Medieval Folklore: A Guide to Myths, Legends, Tales, Beliefs and Customs*, edited by Carl Lindahl, John McNamara and John Lindow. New York: Oxford University Press.

Chen, Nancy. 2008. *Food, Medicine, and the Quest for Good Health: Nutrition, Medicine, and Culture*. New York: Columbia University Press.

Clericuzio, Antonio. 2012. 'Chemical and mechanical theories of digestion in early modern medicine'. *Studies in History and Philosophy of Biological and Biomedical Sciences* 43: 329-337.

Counihan, Carole M. 1999. *The Anthropology of Food and the Body: Gender, Meaning, and Power*. New York: Routledge.

Cramer, J.S., and L.H. Lumey. 2010. 'Maternal Preconception Diet and the Sex Ratio'. *Human Biology* 82 (1): 103-107.

Crocker, Holly A., ed. 2006. *Comic Provocations: Exposing the Corpus of Old French Fabliaux*. New York: Palgrave MacMillan.

Da Soller, Claudio. 2010. 'Beauty, Evolution, and Medieval Literature'. *Philosophy and Literature* 34 (1): 95-111.

Daunay, Marie-Christine, Jules Janick, and Harry S. Paris. 2009. '*Tacuinum sanitatis*: Horticulture and Health in the Late Middle Ages'. *Chronica Horticulturae* 49 (3).

DeVault, Marjorie L. 1991. *Feeding the Family: The Social Organization of Caring as Gendered Work*. Chicago: University of Chicago Press.

Douglas, Mary. 1975. 'Deciphering a Meal'. In *Implicit Meanings: Essays in Anthropology*, edited by Mary Douglas, 248-275. New York: Routledge.

Douglas, Mary. 1996. *Natural Symbols: Explorations in Cosmology*. Second ed. New York: Routledge.

Drabkin, I. E. 1951. 'Soranus and His System of Medicine'. *Bulletin of the History of Medicine* 25 (6): 503-518.

Dubin, Nathaniel E. 2013. *The Fabliaux: A New Verse Translation*. New York: Liveright Publishing Corp.

Dufour, Darna L., Alan H. Goodman, and Gretel Pelto, eds. 2013. *Nutritional Anthropology: Biocultural Perspectives on Food and Nutrition*. Second ed. New York: Oxford University Press.

Dumas, Geneviève. 1996. 'Les femmes et les practiques de la santé dans le "Registre des plaidoiries du Parlement de Paris 1364-1427".' *Canadian Bulletin of Medical History* 13: 13-27.

Dyer, D. J. 2009. 'Gardens and Garden Produce in the Later Middle Ages'. In *Food in Medieval England: Diet and Nutrition*, edited by C.M. Woolgar, D. Serjeantson and T. Waldron, 27-40. New York: Oxford University Press.

Effros, Bonnie. 2002. *Creating Community with Food and Drink in Merovingian Gaul*. New York: Palgrave MacMillan.

Epurescu-Pascovici, Ionut. 2012. 'From Moral Agent to Actant: Conduct in *Le Ménagier de Paris*'. *Exemplaria* 24 (3): 214-37.

Espi-Forcen, Fernando. 2012. 'Anorexia Mirabilis: The Practice of Fasting by Saint Catherine of Siena in the Late Middle Ages'. *American Journal of Psychiatry* 130 (4): 370-371.

Evans, Jennifer. 2014. *Aphrodisiacs, Fertility and Medicine in Early Modern England*. Woodbridge, Suffolk, UK: The Boydell Press for The Royal Historical Society.

Everett, Nicholas, ed. 2014. *The Alphabet of Galen: Pharmacy from Antiquity to the Middle Ages*. Toronto: University of Toronto Press.

Faraone, Christopher A. 2011. 'Magical and Medical Approaches to the Wandering Womb in the Ancient Greek World'. *Classical Antiquity* 30 (1): 1-32.

FDA. 2018. 'Medical Professionals Fast Facts from Food Safety for Moms to Be'. U.S. Food and Drug Adminstration, accessed 10 February 2019. https://www.fda.gov/Food/FoodborneIllnessContaminants/PeopleAtRisk/ucm091671.htm.

Ferrières, Madeleine. 2007. *Nourritures canailles*. Paris: Éditions du Seuil.

Fife, Austin E. 1976. 'Birthmarks and Psychic Imprinting of Babies in Utah Folk Medicine'. In *American Folk Medicine: A Symposium*, edited by Wayland D. Hand, 273-283. Berkeley: University of California Press.

Fissell, Mary. 2004. *Vernacular Bodies: The Politics of Reproduction in Early Modern England*. New York: Oxford University Press.

Fissell, Mary. 2008. 'Introduction: Women, Health, and Healing in Early Modern Europe'. *Bulletin of the History of Medicine* 82:1-17.

Forbes, Thomas R. 1976. 'The Madstone'. In *American Folk Medicine: A Symposium*, edited by Wayland D. Hand, 11-19. Berkeley: University of California Press.

Fox, Robin. 2014. 'Food and Eating: An Anthropological Perspective'. SIRC (Social Issues Research Centre), accessed 2 December 2018. http://www.sirc.org/publik/food_and_eating_0.html.

Frazer, James George. 1999 [1895]. 'The Principles of Sympathetic Magic'. In *International Folkloristics: Classic Contributions by the Founders of Folklore*, edited by Alan Dundas, 109-118. Lanham, MD: Rowman & Littlefield.

Freedman, Paul, and Françoise Marin. 1992. 'Sainteté et sauvagerie: Deux images du paysan au Moyen Age'. *Annales. Histoire, Sciences Sociales* 47 (3): 539-560.

Garay, Kathleen, and Madeleine Jeay, eds. 2006. *The Distaff Gospels: A First Modern English Edition of Les Evangiles Des Quenouilles*. Toronto: The Broadview Press.

Garay, Kathleen, and Madeleine Jeay. 2007. 'Advice Concerning Pregnancy and Health in Late Medieval Europe: Peasant Women's Wisdom in The Distaff Gospels'. *CBMH/BCHM* 23 (2): 423-443.

Gates, Laura Doyle. 1997. 'Distaff and Pen: Producing the *Evangiles des Quenouilles*." *Neophilologus* 81:13-20.

Gaynes, Robert. 2011. *Germ Theory: Medical Pioneers in Infectious Diseases*. Washington, D.C.: ASM Press.

Gazin-Schwartz, Amy, and Cornelius J. Holtorf, eds. 1999. *Archaeology and Folklore*. London: Routledge.

Gentilcore, David. 2004. 'Was there a "Popular Medicine" in Early Modern Europe?' *Folklore* 115 (2):151-166.

Gentilcore, David. 2015. *Food and Health in Early Modern Europe: Diet, Medicine, and Society 1450-1800*. New York: Bloomsbury Academic.

Gérard-Sai, Marie-Claire. 2012. 'Nourrir les seins mercenaires au Moyen Âge'. In *Art de manger, art de vivre: Nourriture et société de l'Antiquité à nos jours*, edited by Veronique Dasen and Marie-Claire Gérard-Zai, 87-102. Gollion, Switzerland: Infolio.

Gilchrist, Roberta. 1999. *Gender and Archeology: Contesting the Past*. New York: Routledge.

Gilchrist, Roberta. 2012. *Archeology and the Life Course*. Woodbridge, UK: The Boydell Press.

Ginzburg, Carlo. 1992 [1980]. *The Cheese and the Worms: The Cosmos of a Sixteenth-Century Miller*. Translated by John Tedeschi and Anne Tedeschi. Baltimore: Johns Hopkins University Press.

Gladwell, Malcolm. 2013 [1998]. 'The Pima Paradox'. In *Nutritional Anthropology: Biocultural Perspectives on Food and Nutrition*, edited by Darna L. Dufour, Alan H. Goodman and Gretel Pelto, 467-478. New York: Oxford University Press.

Glassie, Henry. 1995. 'Tradition'. *Journal of American Folklore* 108 (430): 395-412.

Goodman, Michael K., Josée Johnston, and Kate Cairns. 2017. 'Food, Media and Space: The Mediated Biopolitics of Eating'. *Geoforum* 84:161-168.

Gordon, Sarah. 2007. *Culinary Comedy in Medieval French Literature*. West Lafayette, IN: Purdue University Press.

Gordon, Sarah. 2008. 'Sausages, Nuts, and Eggs: Food Imagery, the Body and Sexuality in the Old French *Fabliaux*'. In *Sexuality in the Middle Ages and the Early Modern Times: New Approaches to a Fundamental Cultural-Historical and Literary-Anthropological Theme*, edited by Albrecht Classen, 503-516. New York: Walter de Gruyter.

Grant, Mark. 2000. *Galen on Food and Diet*. New York: Taylor and Francis.

Greco, Gina L., and Christine M. Rose, eds. 2009. *The Good Wife's Guide: Le Ménagier de Paris, A Medieval Household Book*. Ithaca, NY: Cornell University Press.

Green, Monica H. 2000a. 'Appendix: Medieval Gynecological Literature: A Handlist'. In *Women's Healthcare in the Medieval West: Texts and Contexts*, 1-36. Burlington, VT: Ashgate Variorum.

Green, Monica H. 2000b. 'From "Diseases of Women" to "Secrets of Women": The Transformation of Gynecological Literature in the Later Middle Ages'. *Journal of Medieval and Early Modern Studies* 30 (1): 5-39.

Green, Monica H. 2000c. *Women's Healthcare in the Medieval West: Texts and Contexts*. Burlington, VT: Ashgate.

Green, Monica H., ed. 2002. *The Trotula: An English Translation of the Medieval Compendium of Women's Medicine*. Philadelphia: University of Pennsylvania Press.

Green, Monica H. 2008. *Making Women's Medicine Masculine: The Rise of Male Authority in Pre-Modern Gynaecology*. New York: Oxford University Press.

Greenville, Jane. 2000. 'Houses and Housholds in Late Medieval England: An Archeological Perspective'. In *Medieval Women: Texts and Contexts in Late Medieval Britain – Essays for Felicity Riddy*, edited by Jocelyn Wogan-Browne, Rosalynn Voaden, Arlyn Diamond, Carole Meale Hutchinson, and Lesley Johnson, 309-328. Turnhout: Brepols.

Grimm, Veronika. 1996. *From Feasting to Fasting, the Evolution of a Sin: Attitudes to Food in Late Antiquity*. New York: Routledge.

Halpern, Jennifer. 1982. 'The Infant Formula Debate'. *Food Policy* 7 (1): 85-91.

Hanawalt, Barbara A. 1986. *The Ties That Bound: Peasant Families in Medieval England*. New York: Oxford University Press.

Hand, Wayland D., ed. 1976. *American Folk Medicine: A Symposium*. Berkeley: University of California Press.

Hanson, Anne Ellis. 1975. 'Hippocrates: Diseases of Women 1'. *Signs: Journal of Women in Culture and Society* 1 (2): 567-584.

Harley, David. 1990. 'Historians as Demonologists: The Myth of the Midwife-witch'. *Social History of Medecine* 3 (1): 1-26.

Harris, Marvin. 1998 [1985]. *Good to Eat: Riddles of Food and Culture*. Long Grove, IL: Waveland Press.

Harris-Stoertz, Fiona. 2014. 'Midwives in the Middle Ages? Birth Attendants, 600-1300'. In *Medicine and the Law in the Middle Ages*, edited by Wendy J. Turner and Sara M. Butler, 58-87. Leiden: Brill.

Henisch, Bridget. 1990 [1976]. *Fast and Feast: Food in Medieval Society*. Philadelphia: University of Pennsylvania Press.

Henisch, Bridget. 1995. 'Winter Comforts: Cooking Scenes in Medieval Calendars'. *Petits Propos Culinaires* 50: 25-33.

Hilton, Chadwick B. 1986. 'The Old English "Seasons for Fasting": Its Place in the Vernacular Complaint Tradition'. *Neophilologus* 70 (1):155-159.

Jacquart, Danielle. 2006. 'La nourriture et le corps au Moyen Age'. *Cahiers de recherches médiévales et humanistes* 13 spécial: 259-266.

Jarcho, Saul. 1970. 'Galen's Six Non-Naturals: A Bibliographic Note and Translation'. *Bulletin of the History of Medicine* 44 (4): 372-377.

Jeay, Madeleine. 1982. *Savoir Faire: Une analyse des croyances des 'Evangiles des Quenouilles' (XVe Siècle)*. Montréal: Editions CERES.

Jones, Michael Owen. 2007. 'Food Choice, Symbolism, and Identity: Bread and Butter Issues for Folkloristics and Nutrition Studies (American Folklore Society Presidential Address, October 2005)'. *Journal of American Folklore* 120 (476):129-177.

Jones, Peter. 2019. 'Generation to Reproduction: *The Sekenesse of Wymmen*'. University of Cambridge, accessed 30 November 2019. https://www.reproduction.group.cam.ac.uk/features/sekenesse-of-wymmen.

Karamanou, Marianna, Gregory Tsoucalas, George Creatsas, and George Androutsos. 2013. 'The Effect of Soranus of Ephesus (98-138) on the Work of Midwives." *Women and Birth* 26: 226-228.

Kernan, Sarah Peters. 2015. 'Medieval Cookery Rolls as Practical Kitchen Texts'. *The Recipes Project: Food, Magic, Art, Science, and Medicine*, accessed 5 December 5 2018. http://recipes.hypotheses.org/tag/cookery-books.

King, Helen. 2007. *Midwifery, Obstetrics and the Rise of Gynaecology: The Uses of a Sixteenth-Century Compendium*. Burlington, VT: Ashgate.

Kingston, Rosari. 2017. 'Folk Medicine and Its Second Life'. *Estudios Irelandeses* 12: 91-106.

Kitta, Andrea. 2018. 'Alternative Health Websites and Fake News: Taking a Stab at Definition, Genre, and Belief'. *Journal of American Folklore* 131 (522): 405-412.

Klein, Jakob, and James L. Watson, eds. 2016. *The Handbook of Food and Anthropology*. New York: Bloomsbury Academic.

Klemettilä, Hannele. 2012. *The Medieval Kitchen: A Social History with Recipes*. London: Reaktion Books.

Knight, Alan E. 1983. 'The Condemnation of Pleasure in Late Medieval French Morality Plays'. *The French Review* 57 (1): 1-9.

Kroeber, Alfred L. 1987 [1952]. 'The Nature of Culture'. In *Perspectives in Cultural Anthropology*, edited by Herbert Applebaum, 80-84. Albany: SUNY Press.

Krueger, Roberta L. 2005. 'Identity Begins at Home: Female Conduct and the Failure of Counsel in *Le Ménagier de Paris*'. *Essays in Medieval Studies* 22: 21-39.

Kyle, Sarah R. 2017. *Medicine and Humanism in Late Medieval Italy: The Carrara Herbal in Padua*. New York: Routledge.

Langland, William. 2006. *Piers Plowman, Norton Critical Editions*. New York: W.W. Norton.

Laudun, Rachel. 2013. *Cuisine and Empire: Cooking in World History*. Berkeley: University of California Press.

Laurent, Sylvie. 1989. *Naître au Moyen Age: de la conception à la naissance: la grossese et l'accouchement*. Paris: Le Léopard d'Or.

Laurioux, Bruno. 2002. *Manger au Moyen Âge: Pratiques et discours alimentaires en Europe aux XVIe et XVe siècles*. Paris: HACHETTE Littératures.

Laurioux, Bruno. 2006a. 'Cuisine et médecine au Moyen Âge: Alliés ou ennemies?' *Cahiers de recherches médiévales et humanistes* 13 spécial: 223-238.

Laurioux, Bruno. 2006b. *Gastronomie, humanisme et société à Rome au milieu du XVe siècle: Autour du De honesta voluptate de Platina*. Firenze: Edizioni de Galluzzo.

Laurioux, Bruno. 2011. *Écrits et images de la gastronomie médiévale*. Paris: Bibliothèque nationale de France.

Leatherman, Thomas L., and Alan H. Goodman. 2013 [2005]. 'Coca-Colonization of Diets in the Yucatán'. In *Nutritional Anthropology: Biocultural Perpectives on Food and Nutrition*, edited by Darna L. Dufour, Alan H. Goodman and Gretel Pelto, 383-395. New York: Oxford University Press.

Lelwica, Michelle. 2006. Redefining Womanhood (?): Gender, Power, and the "Religion of Thinness". *Anthropology of Food* 5.

Lemay, Helen Rodnite. 1992. *Women's Secrets: A Translation of Pseudo-Albertus Magnus's De Secretis Mulierum with Commentaries*. Edited by Paul E. Szarmach, *SUNY Series in Medieval Studies*. Albany: SUNY Press.

Levenstein, Harvey. 2003. *Revolution at the Table: The Transformation of the American Diet.* Berkeley: University of California Press.

Lévi-Strauss, Claude. 1966. 'The Culinary Triangle'. *Partisan Review* 33: 586-595.

Lévi-Strauss, Claude. 1983 [1969]. *The Raw and the Cooked.* Translated by John Weightman and Doreen Weightman, *Mythologiques.* Chicago: University of Chicago Press.

Li, Ching-Chu, Kan-Lin Hsu, Chih-Hsuan Chen, and Bih-Ching Shu. 2017. 'The Impact of Traditional Health Beliefs on the Health Practices of Women from Southern Taiwan'. *Journal of Transcultural Nursing* 28 (5): 473-478.

Lindow, John. 2018. 'The Challenge of Folklore to Medieval Studies'. *Humanities* 7 (15) :5.

Lochrie, Karma. 2016. *Nowhere in the Middle Ages.* Philadephia: University of Pennsylvania Press.

Long, Lucy M. 2009. 'Introduction'. *Journal of American Folklore* 122 (483):1-13.

Long, Lucy M., ed. 2015. *The Food and Folklore Reader.* New York: Bloomsbury Academic.

Lozinski, Grégoire. 1933. *La Bataille de Caresme et de Charnage: édition critique avec introduction glossaire.* Paris: Librairie Ancienne Honoré Champion.

Lysaght, Patricia. 1994. 'Women, Milk and Magic at the Boundary Festival of May'. In *Milk and Milk Products from Medieval to Modern Times: Proceedings of the Ninth International Conference on Ethnological Food Research, Ireland, 1992,* edited by Patricia Lysaght, 208-229. Edinburgh: Canongate Press.

Majeed, Azeem. 2005. 'How Islam Changed Medicine: Arab Physicians and Scholars Laid the Basis for Medical Practice in Europe'. *British Medical Journal* 331 (7531): 1486-1487.

Marafioti, Martin. 2010. 'The Prescriptive Potency in Michele Savonarola's *De Regimine Pregnantium*'. In *Table Talk: Perspectives on Food in Medieval Italian Literature,* edited by Christina Purdy Moudarres, 19-33. Newcastle upon Tyne: Cambridge Scholars Publishing.

Marcos-Marín, Francisco. 1999. 'Masculine Beauty vs. Feminine Beauty in Medieval Iberia'. In *Multicultural Iberia: Language, Literature, and Music,* edited by Dru Dougherty and Milton M. Azevado, 22-39. Berkeley: University of California.

Markham, Gervais. 1986 [1615]. *The English Housewife.* Edited by Michael R. Best. Montreal: McGill-Queen's University Press.

Marquez, Mary N., and Consualo Pacheco. 1964. 'Midwifery Lore in New Mexico'. *The American Journal of Nursing* 64 (9): 81-84.

Marron, Brianna M. 2014. 'A Space of Convergence: Hildegard of Bingen's Multivalent Understanding of the Body'. *Magistra* 20 (2): 38-57.

Martin, A. Lynn. 2009. *Alcohol, Violence, and Disorder in Traditional Europe*. Kirksville, MO: Truman State University Press.

Marty-Dufaut, Josy. 2016. *Cuisiniers et ouvrages culinaires du Moyen Âge: Au coeur de la cuisine médiévale*. Rennes, France: éditions Ouest-France.

Matalas, Antonia-Leda, Antonis Zampelas, and Vassilis Stavrinos. 2001. *The Mediterranean Diet: Constituants and Health Promotion*. Boca Raton, FL: CRC Press.

McIntosh, W. Alex, and Mary Zey. 1989. 'Women as Gatekeepers of Food Consumption: A Sociological Critique'. *Food and Foodways* 3 (4): 317-332.

McNaughton, Darlene. 2011. 'From the Womb to the Tomb: Obesity and Maternal Responsibility'. In *Alcohol, Tobacco and Obesity: Morality, Mortality and the New Public Health*, edited by Kirsten Bell, Amy Salmon and Darlene McNaughton, 163-176. New York: Routledge.

Meyer-Rochow, Victor Benno. 2009. 'Food Taboos: Their Origins and Purposes'. *Journal of Enthobiology and Ethnomedicine* 5 (18).

Micke, Oliver, and Jutta Hübner. 2009. 'Traditional European Medicine – After all, is Hildegard von Bingen really right?' *European Journal of Integrative Medicine* 1 (4): 226.

Milham, Mary Ella. 1998. *Platina: On Right Pleasure and Good Health; A Critical Edition and Translation of De honesta voluptate et valetudine*. Tempe, AZ: Medieval and Renaissance Texts and Studies.

Minkowsky, William L. 1992. 'Women Healers of the Middle Ages: Selected Aspects of their History'. *American Journal of Public Health* 82 (2): 288-295.

Mintz, Sidney W. 1985. *Sweetness and Power: The Place of Sugar in Modern History*. New York: Viking.

Mintz, Sidney W., and Christine M. Du Bois. 2002. 'The Anthropology of Food and Eating'. *Annual Review of Anthropology* 31: 99-119.

Montanari, Massimo. 2012. *Medieval Tastes: Food, Cooking, and the Table*. Translated by Beth Archer Brombert. New York: Columbia University Press.

Monti, Davorka. 2000. 'Food Customs and their Role in Pregnancy and Infant Feeding'. *International Journal of Childbirth Education* 15 (4):18.

Mormiche, Pascale, and Stanis Perez, eds. 2016. *Naissance et petite enfance à la cour de France: Moyen Age-XIXe siècle*. Villeneuve d'Ascq, France: Presses universitaires du Septentrion.

Mukhopadhyay, Susmita, and Arpita Sarkar. 2009. 'Pregnancy-related food habits among women of rural Sikkim, India'. *Public Health Nutrition* 12 (12): 2317-2322.

Müldner, Gundula, and Michael P. Richards. 2005. 'Fast or Feast: Reconstructing Diet in Later Medieval England by Stable Isotope Analysis'. *Journal of Archeological Science* 32 (1): 39-48.

Musacchio, Jaqueline Marie. 1999. *The Art and Ritual of Childbirth in Renaissance Italy*. New Haven: Yale University Press.

Nabinger, Laurieanne. 2019. 'Managing Pain with Traditional Chinese Medicine'. Veteran's Administration Puget Sound Health Care System, accessed 30 November 2019. https://www.va.gov/PAINMANAGEMENT/Veteran_Public/Veteran_docs/TRADITIONAL-CHINESE-MEDICINE-Booklet.pdf.

Nichter, Mark, and Mimi Nichter. 1983. 'Ethnophysiology and Folk Dietetics of Pregnancy: A Case Study from South India'. *Human Organization* 42 (3): 235-247.

Nicoud, Marilyn. 2006. 'Savoirs et pratiques diététiques au Moyen Âge'. *Cahiers de recherches médiévales et humanistes* (13 spécial).

Nicoud, Marilyn. 2008. "Food Consumption, A Health Risk? Norms and Medical Practice in the Middle Ages'. *Appetite* (51): 7-9.

Nilden-Wall, Bodil, and Jan Wall. 1993. 'The Witch as Hare or the Witch's Hare: Popular Legends and Beliefs in Nordic Tradition'. *Folklore* 104 (1/2): 67-76.

Notaker, Henry. 2017. *A History of Cookbooks: From Kitchen to Page over Seven Centuries*. Berkeley: University of California Press.

O'Connor, Bonnie B., and David J. Hufford. 2001. 'Understanding Folk Medicine'. In *Healing Logics: Culture and Medicine in Modern Health Belief Systems*, edited by Erika Brady, 13-35. Logan, UT: Utah State University Press.

O'Dea, Karin. 1984. 'Marked Improvement in Carbohydrate and Lipid Metabolism in Diabetic Australian Aborigines After Temporary Reversion to Traditional Lifestyle'. *Diabetes* 33 (6): 596-603.

Parkhurst-Ferguson, Priscilla. 2004. *Accounting for Taste: The Triumph of French Cuisine*. Chicago: University of Chicago Press.

Passmore, S. Elizabeth, and Susan Carter, eds. 2007. *The English 'Loathly Lady' Tales: Boundaries, Traditions, Motifs*. Kalamazoo, MI: Medieval Institute Publications.

Payen, Jean-Charles. 1981. 'Fabliaux et Cocagne: Abondance et fête charnelle dans les contes plaisants du XIIe et du XIIIe siècles'. Epopée animale, fable, fabliau: acts du IVe colloque de la Société internationale renardienne, Evreux, France.

Pearce, John M. S. 2008. 'The Doctrine of Signatures'. *European Neurology* 60: 51-52.

Penn State. 2015. ' "To beet or not to beet?" Researchers test theories of beet juice benefits'. accessed 30 November 2019. https://www.sciencedaily.com/releases/2015/01/150119083300.htm.

Pernoud, Régine. 1998. *Women in the Days of the Cathedrals*. Translated by Anne Coté-Harriss. San Francisco: Ignatius Press.

Pillsbury, Barbara L.K. 1978. "Doing the Month: Confinement and Convalescence of Chinese Women after Childbirth'. *Medical Anthropology* 12:11-22.

Piper, Leanne. 2010. 'The Professionalization of Midwifery in the Late Middle Ages'. *Canadian Journal of Midwifery Research and Practice* 9 (1): 21-34.

Poor, Sara S., and Jana K. Schulman, eds. 2007. *Women and Medieval Epic: Gender, Genre, and the Limits of Epic Masculinity.* Basingstoke, UK: Palgrave MacMillan.

Quave, Cassandra L., Manual Pardo-de-Santayana, and Andrea Pieroni. 2012. 'Medical Ethnobotony in Europe: From Field Ethnography to a More Culturally Sensitive Evidence-Based CAM?' *Evidence-Based Complementary and Alternative Medicine* Special Issue.

Rasmussen, Kathleen M., and Ann L. Yaktine, eds. 2009. *Weight Gain During Pregnancy: Reexamining the Guidelines.* Washington, D.C.: National Academies Press.

Rawcliffe, Carole. 2008. 'Rooted in the Earth, Rooted in the Sky: Hildegard of Bingen and Premodern Medicine by Victoria Sweet (review)'. *Speculum* 83 (3): 766-767.

Redon, Odile, Françoise Sabban, and Silvano Serventi. 1998 [1991]. *The Medieval Kitchen: Recipes from France and Italy.* Translated by Edward Schneider. Chicago: University of Chicago Press.

Reischer, Erica, and Kathryn S. Koo. 2004. 'The Body Beautiful: Symbolism and Agency in the Social World'. *Annual Review of Anthropology* 33: 297-317.

Retief, Francois P., and Louise C. Cilliers. 2001. 'The Influence of Christianity on Graeco-Roman Medicine Up to the Renaissance'. *Akroterion* 46: 6-73.

Retief, Francois P., and Louise C. Cilliers. 2010. 'Astrology and Medicine in Antiquity and the Middle Ages'. *South African Journal of Science and Technology* 29 (1):1-9.

Riddle, John M. 2013. 'Folk Tradition and Folk Medicine: Recognition of Drugs in Classical Antiquity'. *Pharmacy in History* 55 (2/3): 64-87.

Rigby, Stephen H. 2000. 'The Wife of Bath, Christine de Pizan, and the Medieval Case for Women'. *The Chaucer Review* 35 (2): 133-165.

Ritchey, Sara. 2014. 'Affective Medicine: Later Medieval Healing Communities and the Feminization of Health Care Practices in the Thirteenth-Century Low Countries'. *Journal of Medieval Religious Cultures* 40 (2): 113-143.

Rose, Christine M. 2002. 'What Every Goodwoman Wants: The Parameters of Desire in *Le Ménagier de Paris/ The Goodman of Paris*'. *Studia Anglica Posnaniensia* 38: 393-410.

Rowland, Beryl. 1981. *Medieval Woman's Guide to Health: The First English Gynecological Handbook.* Kent, OH: Kent State University Press.

Rowley, Anthony. 2006. *Une histoire mondiale de la table: Stratégies de bouche.* Paris: Odile Jacob.

Saguy, Abigail C., and Kjerstin Gruys. 2010. 'Morality and Health: News Media Constructions of Overweight and Eating Disorders'. *Social Problems* 57 (2).

Salomonsson, Anders. 1994. 'Milk and Folk Belief: With Examples from Sweden'. In *Milk and Milk Products from Medieval to Modern Times: Proceedings of the Ninth International Conference on Ethnological Food Research, Ireland, 1992*, edited by Patricia Lysaght, 191-197. Edinburgh: Canongate Press.

Santacroce, Luigi, Lucrezia Bottalico, and Ioannis Alexandros Charitos. 2017. 'Greek Medicine Practice at Ancient Rome: The Physician Molecularist Asclepiades'. *Medicines (Basel)* 4 (4): 92-99.

Scappi, Bartolomeo. 2011 [1570]. *The Opera of Bartolomeo Scappi: The Art and Craft of a Master Cook*. Translated by Terence Scully. Toronto: University of Toronto Press.

Scarborough, Peter, Prachi Bhatnagar, Kremlin K. Wickramasinghe, Steve Allender, Charlie Foster, and Mike Rayner. 2011. 'The economic burden of ill health due to diet, physical inactivity, smoking, alcohol and obesity in the UK: an update to 2006-07 NHS costs'. *Journal of Public Health* 33 (4): 527-535.

Schmitt, Jean-Claude. 1998. 'Religion, Folklore, and Society in the Medieval West'. In *Debating the Middle Ages: Issues and Readings*, edited by Lester K. Little and Barbara H. Rosenwein, 378-87. Oxford: Blackwell.

Schulman, Jana K. 2007. ' "A Guest in the Hall": Women, Feasts, and Violence in Icelandic Epic'. In *Women and Medieval Epic: Gender, Genre, and the Limits of Epic Masculinity*, edited by Sara S. Poor and Jana K. Schulman, 209-233. Basingstoke, UK: Palgrave MacMillan.

Scully, Terence. 1995. *The Art of Cookery in the Middle Ages*. Rochester, NY: The Boydell Press.

Shapiro, Laura. 2001. *Perfection Salad: Women and Cooking at the Turn of the Century*. New York: The Modern Library.

Shuffleton, George. 2008. 'How the Good Wife Taught her Daughter--Introduction'. *TEAMS Middle English Texts Series*, accessed 1 August 2018. http://d.lib.rochester.edu/teams/text/shuffelton-codex-ashmole-61-how-the-good-wife-taught-her-daughter-introduction.

Shukla, Pravina. 2008. *The Grace of the Four Moons: Dress, Adornment, and the Art of the Body in Modern India*. Bloomington: Indiana University Press.

Siraisi, Nancy G. 2009. *Medieval and Early Renaissance Medicine: An Introduction to Knowledge and Practice*. Chicago: University of Chicago Press.

Skelton, John. 2011 [1550]. *The Tunning of Elinor Rumming: A Poem*. London: Eighteenth Century Collections Online Print Editions. Original edition, Isaac Dalton for W. Boreham.

Small, Meredith. 1999. 'A Woman's Curse'. *Sciences* 39 (1): 24-29.

Smith, Sally V. 2007a. 'Women and Power in the Late Medieval English Village: A Reconsideration'. *Women's History Review* 16 (3): 311-321.

Smith, William Bradford. 2007b. 'Food and Deception in the Discourse on Heresy and Witchcraft in Bamburg'. In *At the Table: Metaphorical and Material Cultures of Food in Medieval and Early Modern Europe*, edited by Timothy J. Tomasik and Juliann M. Vitullo, 107-122. Turnhout: Brepols.

Sneath, David. 2018. 'From Transactionalism to Practice Theory'. In *Schools and Styles of Anthropological Theory*, edited by Candea Matei, 91-107. New York: Routledge.

Stannard, Jerry. 2013. 'Medieval Herbalism and Post-Medieval Folk Medicine'. *Pharmacy in History* 55 (2/3): 47-54.

Stearns, Peter N. 2002. *Fat History: Bodies and Beauty in the Modern West*. Second ed. New York: New York University Press.

Stelmack, Robert M., and Anistasios Stalikos. 1991. 'Galen and the Humour Theory of Temperament'. *Personality and Individual Differences* 12 (3): 255-263.

Stoeckle, John. 1984. 'Medical Advice Books: The Search for the Healthy Body'. *Social Science & Medicine* 18 (9): 707-712.

Stolberg, Michael. 2012. ' "Abhorreas pinguedinem": Fat and obesity in early modern medicine (c. 1500-1750)'. *Studies in History and Philosophy of Biological and Biomedical Sciences* 43: 370-378.

Strathern, Andrew J. 1996. *Body Thoughts*. Ann Arbor: University of Michigan Press.

Stuard, Susan Mosher. 1975. 'Dame Trot'. *Signs: Journal of Women in Culture and Society* 1 (2): 537-452.

Stuard, Susan Mosher. 2007. 'Rooted in the Earth, Rooted in the Sky: Hildegard of Bingen and Premodern Medicine (review)'. *Journal of the History of Medicine and Allied Sciences* 62 (3): 359-361.

Sweet, Victoria. 1999. 'Hildegard of Bingen and the Greening of Medieval Medicine'. *Bulletin of the History of Medicine* 73 (3): 381-403.

Sweet, Victoria. 2006. *Rooted in the Earth, Rooted in the Sky: Hildegard of Bingen and Premodern Medicine*. New York: Routledge.

Talbot, Charles H. 1976. 'Folk Medicine and History'. In *American Folk Medicine: A Symposium*, edited by Wayland D. Hand, 7-10. Berkeley: University of California Press.

Tambiah, Stanley J. 2017 [1973]. 'Form and meaning of magical acts: A point of view'. *HAU: Journal of Ethnographic Theory* 3: 451-473.

Tanner, Norman, and Sethina Watson. 2006. 'Least of the Laity: The Minimum Requirements for a Medieval Christian'. *Journal of Medieval History* 32 (4): 395-423.

Tertullian. 2017 [1885]. 'On the Apparel of Women'. New Advent Online Catholic Encyclopedia, accessed 26 June 2018. http://www.newadvent.org/fathers/0402.htm.

Theophano, Janet. 2002. *Eat My Words: Reading Women's Lives through the Cookbooks They Wrote*. New York: Palgrave.

Throop, Priscilla. 2006. 'Introduction'. In *Causes and Cures: The Complete English Translation of Hildegardis Causae et Curae Libri V*, edited by Priscilla Throop. Charlotte, VT: Medieval MS.

Thursby, Jacqueline S. 2008. *Foodways and Folklore: A Handbook*. Westport, CT: Greenwood Press.

Tomasik, Timothy J. 2007. 'Translating Taste in the Vernacular Editions of Platina's *De Honesta Voluptate et Valetudine*'. In *At the Table: Metaphorical and Material Cultures of Food in Medieval and Early Modern Europe*, edited by Timothy J. Tomasik and Juliann M. Vitullo, 189-210. Turnhout: Brepols.

Toulalan, Sarah. 2014. ' "To[o] much eating stifles the child": Fat Bodies and Reproduction in Early Modern England'. *Historical Research* 87 (235): 65-93.

Toulalan, Sarah. 2017. ' "If slendernesse be the cause of unfruitfulnesse; you must nourish and fatten the body"; Thin Bodies and Infertility in Early Modern England'. In *The Palgrave Handbook of Infertility in History: Approaches, Contexts and Perspectives*, edited by Gayle Davis and Tracey Loughran, 171-197. London: Palgrave Macmillan.

Tye, Diane. 2010. *Baking as Biography: A Life Story in Recipes*. Kingston, ON: McGill-Queen's University Press.

U.S. National Library of Medicine. 2011. 'Islamic Culture and the Medical Arts: The Great Systematizers'. National Institutes of Health, accessed 11 November 2017. https://www.nlm.nih.gov/exhibition/islamic_medical/islamic_07.html.

Udry, Susan. 2002. 'Robert de Blois and Geoffroy de la Tour Landry on Feminine Beauty: Two Late Medieval French Conduct Books for Women'. *Essays in Medieval Studies* 19: 90-102.

UNFAO. 2013. *FAO Policy on Gender Equality: Attaining Food Security Goals in Agriculture and Rural Development*. Rome: Food and Agriculture Organization of the United Nations.

van Winter, Johanna Maria. 2007. *Spices and Comfits: Collected Papers on Medieval Food*. Totnes, Devon: Prospect Books.

Vaughan, Theresa A. 2011. "The Alewife: Changing Images and Bad Brews." *AVISTA: Studies in the History of Medieval Science, Technology, and Art* 21 (1/2): 34-41.

Vaughan, Theresa A. 2014. ' "Composed for the honor and glory of the Ladies": Folklore and Medieval Women's Sexuality in the *Distaff Gospels*'. In *Unsettling Assumptions: Tradition, Gender, Drag*, edited by Pauline Greenhill and Diane Tye, 208-225. Logan, UT: Utah State University Press.

Vigarello, Georges. 1993. *Histoire des pratiques de santé: Le sain et le malsain depuis le Moyen Âge*. Paris: Éditions du Seuil.

Vigarello, Georges. 2010. *Les métamorphoses du gras: Histoire de l'obésité du Moyen Âge au XXe siècle*. Paris: Éditions du Seuil.

Vitale, Lisa. 2010. 'Deprivation and Fullness: The Dietary Dialectics of St. Catherine of Sienna'. In *Table Talk: Perspectives on Food in Medieval Italian Literature*, edited by Christina Purdy Moudarres, 53-69. Newcastle upon Tyne: Cambridge Scholars Publishing.

Waines, David 1999. 'Dietetics in Medieval Islamic Culture'. *Medical History* 43: 228-240.

Wallis, Faith, ed. 2010. *Medieval Medicine: A Reader*. Toronto: University of Toronto Press.

Watts, Sydney. 2012. 'Food and the Annales School'. In *The Oxford Handbook of Food History*, edited by Jeffrey M. Pilcher, 3-22. New York: Oxford University Press.

Weber, A.S. 1998. 'Queu du Roi, Roi des Queux: Taillevent and the Profession of Medieval Cooking'. In *Food and Eating in Medieval Europe*, edited by Martha Carlin and Joel T. Rosenthal, 145-158. London: The Hambledon Press.

Wein-Plus. 2018. 'Heunisch'. accessed 27 November 2018. https://glossary.wein-plus.eu/heunisch.

Weiss-Amer, Melitta. 1992. 'Dietetics of Pregnancy: A Fifteenth-Century Perspective'. *Fifteenth Century Studies* 19: 301-318.

Weiss-Amer, Melitta. 1993. 'Medieval Women's Guides to Food during Pregnancy: Origins, Texts, and Traditions'. *Canadian Bulletin of Medical History* 10: 5-23.

Wells, Sharon. 2002. 'Food in the City: An Interdisciplinary Study of the Ideological and Symbolic Uses of Food in the Urban Environment in Later Medieval England'. Ph.D., The Centre for Medieval Studies, University of York.

Wiegelmann. 2015 [1974]. 'Innovations in Food and Meals'. In *The Food and Folklore Reader*, edited by Lucy M. Long, 39-47. New York: Bloomsbury Academic.

Witthoft, Brucia. 1978. 'The *Tacuinum sanititatis*: A Lombard Panorama'. *Gesta* 17 (1): 49-60.

Woolgar, C.M. 2009a. 'Group Diets in Late Medieval England'. In *Food in Medieval England: Diet and Nutrition*, edited by C.M. Woolgar, D. Serjeantson and T. Waldron, 191-200. New York: Oxford University Press.

Woolgar, C.M. 2009b. 'Meat and Dairy Products in Late Medieval England'. In *Food in Medieval England: Diet and Nutrition*, edited by C.M. Woolgar, D. Serjeantson and T. Waldron, 88-101. New York: Oxford University Press.

Woolgar, C.M. 2010. 'Food in the Middle Ages'. *Journal of Medieval History* 36: 1-19.

Woolgar, C.M., D. Serjeantson, and T. Waldron, eds. 2009. *Food in Medieval England: Diet and Nutrition*. New York: Oxford University Press.

Yoder, Don. 1972. 'Folk Cookery'. In *Folklore and Folklife*, edited by Richard Dorson, 334. Chicago: University of Chicago Press.

York, William H. 2012. *Health and Wellness in Antiquity through the Middle Ages*. Santa Barbara: Greenwood Press.

Young, Katherine, ed. 1993. *Bodylore*. Edited by Patrick B. Mullen, *Publications of the American Folklore Society, New Series*. Knoxville: University of Tennessee Press.

Ziment, Irwin. 2002. 'Spices, Exotic Flavors and Medicines: Sugar'. UCLA History and Special Collections Louse M. Darling Biomedical Library, accessed 30 November 2019. https://unitproj.library.ucla.edu/biomed/spice/index.cfm?displayID=23.

Index

For Product Safety Concerns and Information please contact our EU representative GPSR@taylorandfrancis.com
Taylor & Francis Verlag GmbH, Kaufingerstraße 24, 80331 München, Germany

www.ingramcontent.com/pod-product-compliance
Ingram Content Group UK Ltd.
Pitfield, Milton Keynes, MK11 3LW, UK
UKHW022131190926
475702UK00013B/1749
9781041190844